SUFFERING, DEATH, AND IDENTITY

VALUE INQUIRY BOOK SERIES

VIBS

Volume 135

a volume in

Personalist Studies
PS
Steven Schroeder, Editor

SUFFERING, DEATH, AND IDENTITY

Edited by

Robert N. Fisher
Daniel T. Primozic
Peter A. Day
Joel A. Thompson

Rodopi

Amsterdam - New York, NY 2002

The paper on which this book is printed meets the requirements of "ISO 9706:1994, Information and documentation - Paper for documents - Requirements for permanence".

ISBN: 90-420-1173-4

Printed in the Netherlands

CONTENTS

FOREWORD

Personalist Studies is a creative and innovative special series designed to create and promote interdisciplinary and multi-disciplinary dialogue. Instead of remaining within the confines of one subject specialism, the special series actively engages in issues which cut across a wide range of philosophical areas, interests, and concerns.

The call to personhood is the primary challenge of life in the twenty-first century. The challenge to place persons at the heart of all our thinking and living must not be ignored. Now, more than ever, an imperative is at work to explore what it means to be and to become persons in the context of our social, cultural, national, and international relationships. The increasing complexity of daily living, and the rapidly changing scientific and technological revolutions which form the horizons within which such a life is lived, leave little time for a sense of the personal.

To be hoped for is a new type of thinking which emerges from ancient roots—a personalist philosophy—which recognizes the uniqueness of human beings, the fostering of a more humane approach to life, and the need to make sure that our reflections and our conversations are not carried out in the isolating confines of academic life, and in a language only the elite can understand. We must ensure that discussions of the issues which surround persons are open to anyone who wants to join them, and that the implications and consequences which follow from them, have real, practical, outcomes and effects. Personalist Studies aims to provide a forum for such conversations.

Robert N. Fisher

PREFACE

Toward the end of the previous millennium, Oriel College, Oxford, could not display its usual verdant quadrangles. Instead, it could offer its inhabitants and visitors only a burning heat accompanying the "worst drought in five-hundred years" and pale tan lawns. Yet Oxford remained its ancient, inspiring self and graciously became host to the third international *Conference on Persons*.

Scholars gathered from across the world to share their work concerning the nature, lives, and deaths of persons. This concept of persons is at once both plain and technical, difficult to define but easy to use, complex in relationship to other concepts and allegedly simple in scope, broad in its application and precise in meaning, powerful in moral, legal, and emotional ramifications and humble in appearance only. Those participating scholars spent a week discussing crucial human issues both perennial and brand new. They brought their hard-won thoughts to the dry land of England that year to have them scrutinized, criticized, and praised. They were, themselves, persons who maintained wonder at the nobility and frailty of human beings of every kind and at the very idea of personhood. The discussions which took place seared a noble impression upon my memory for two important reasons.

Some of the participants were old hands at the century-old school of thought called "personalism." Some of us had just been introduced to the work of the distinguished American philosopher, Borden Parker Bowne, and the like-minded spirits from around the world that his thinking spawned. Without digressing here into a history of the personalist movement, I will say that those spirits and those of us who attended the conference had one thing in common: the will and the reason to assert and reassert the value of humanity in the face of an ongoing and growing onslaught of modern and contemporary impersonalism. The influence of early personalists and the work of the current proponents of personalism are yours to behold in the pages that follow and, thus, need no further chatter from me. The high quality and significance of their work is manifest and made a lasting impression upon me as it doubtless will upon you.

What is not so available to the readers of this volume is the delightful surprise that the people of the conference not only "talked a good personalist game" but also lived their intellectual commitments as well. They were keen, kind, constructive, helpful, critical, insightful, and a joy to engage. They were a rare philosophical breed who practiced well their preaching, and by their living precedent gave both the movement of personalism and humanity *per se* a hopeful example. Even from their writings we may glean some idea of what I have claimed about their noble, living commitments. Here I will end to let them begin their "celebration of persons."

Daniel T. Primozic

ACKNOWLEDGMENTS

The editors of this book thank all the contributors for the high quality of their work. Special thanks to James Magrini and Joel Huotari for their help in the final edits. Thanks to Elmhurst College and its Center for Professional Excellence for their support both moral and financial. Hearty thanks go to our loved ones for their patience during this project, and to Robert Ginsberg and Steven Schroeder for their expert and dedicated editorial work. Thanks finally to Oriel College, Oxford, for hosting an excellent and productive Conference on Persons. Part of Chapter Nine, "HIV and Religion: Toward a New Dialogue," was published in *Contact, The Interdisciplinary Journal of Pastoral Studies*, 113, 1994, pp. 20-26, and appears here with permission.

One

INTRODUCTION

Robert N. Fisher

Amid the plethora of competing and constantly changing agendas of modern life, one call remains steadfast: the imperative to be and become persons in the context of our social, cultural, national, and international relationships. The chapters in this book have been written with these aims in mind. The focus falls within the boundaries of what happens to persons and to a person's sense of identity when confronted by pain, suffering, and death. Human life is vulnerable to moments or even extended periods of "personal crisis" brought about by physical illness, disease, or disability, as well as the psychological and mental suffering which often accompany these. In such times, a person's identity can be placed under severe stress leading to the breakdown and dissolution of the sense of who we are, and often opening the horizon for the emergence of an altered or new sense of personhood.

The pressure on our identity is not restricted solely to the confines of our own "first-hand" experience of suffering. The suffering, pain, and death of those we love or with whom we share an acquaintance or friendship can act as a trigger to undermine the confidence we have in ourselves as persons. Our awareness of the suffering of others in a national or global context can also raise a sense of disquiet and discomfort with the familiar territory that we call ourselves. The question of human suffering necessarily becomes a question about the complex interpersonal relationships we build and develop; and a person's identity exists in an uneasy state of qualified stability in relation with and in response to all the fluctuating circumstances and events which constitute human life.

Three qualities or elements characterize our encounter with suffering. First, suffering is characterized as an event which disrupts, interrupts, or intrudes into the normal flow or pattern of daily life. Suffering prevents the continuation of the narratives we use to make sense of who we are and the meaning of the life we live. Narrative disintegrates under the burden of suffering. Our sense of identity is left without the normal boundaries which provide security and stability, with the twofold effect that we are left either with a longing for the time before suffering arose, or with the disability of knowing what narrative we can tell in the present. In the immediate aftermath of an event of suffering, we are left bewildered, shocked, numbed, forced into a silence that testifies both to the inability of our previous narratives to make sense of what is happening and to the dawning realization that we do not know what to do, how to react, or even who we are. Silence affirms the loss of confidence in our sense of identity, the breakdown of the structures which gave meaning to our lives, and to the loss of direction in the telling of the story of who we are. The foundations which provide the ability to respond no longer guarantee a sure footing.

Second, suffering requires or imposes self-scrutiny; the processes which give rise to many of the questions we ask partly constitute our suffering. In the absence of narrative, these questions are incapable of finding an answer, but they do reflect a gradual reexamination of our sense of identity in the light of the intrusiveness of what has happened. "Why me?" captures the forlorn gamut of emotions experienced by the person who is suffering—for example, feelings of injustice (I have been a good person—why should this happen to me?), outrage (I do not deserve this), and bewilderment (why has this happened?). Such questions do not require a public answer; instead, they indicate a "losing of the way" a person once thought was sure and certain, a failure to "pick up the plot" that once held the meaning of a life together. The "why?" question is a quizzical groping after the lost sense of self; no answers are required. The best we can offer is a comforting presence, the silent holding of a hand, a warm embrace.

Third, the gradual discovery of a path through suffering, if one is found at all, involves a change of perspective occasioned by the emergence of a new or altered set of narratives. Perhaps the question changes from "why?" to "how?" Now that this has happened, how do I cope? Perhaps a change of emphasis occurs on the questions asked brought about by the passage of time; perhaps the momentum created by external factors necessitates a moving on and a pragmatic demand to live life in spite of or in the continued presence of suffering. Each person finds his or her own way through suffering, but the ability to do so marks an often unconscious shift in the foundations which enable us to respond to the suffering in our lives as well as in relation to the competing demands of those with whom we live. This shift signifies the gradual discovery of a tentatively new sense of self, continuous with the previous sense of identity yet accompanied by a set of narratives which enable the emergence of a radically new and discontinuous exploration of who we are. Suffering sets the tone of our new narratives, and is inextricably bound up with the plot which begins to emerge. We may only be dimly aware of where the new story will lead us; because a new story is being told, though, it testifies to the fundamental change which has taken place in the foundations which shape our identity.

For the observers of suffering, the picture is not necessarily different. To be a witness to the suffering of others indicates two facts. First, that suffering is never isolated. Although the impact of suffering within people creates the feeling of isolation, insularity, and loneliness, their presence within a network of relationships entails that the impact does not remain solely with the sufferers. Suffering is necessarily interpersonal. We suffer with and on behalf of those who are suffering. Their suffering causes and creates suffering in us. No selfishness is involved; nor does any desire exist to avoid the feelings which the suffering of those we love and care for engenders within us—save for the overwhelming wish that things were otherwise for the sufferer. When suffering is seen as an interpersonal experience, the nature of suffering changes as it becomes an event which concerns us all, and which is shaped by the presence of all those who are involved with the sufferer.

The second fact we therefore need to notice is that the suffering of others is a constitutive factor in our own personal identity. The presence of disability, illness, hurt, and anguish in the lives of those around us cannot leave us unaffected. An encounter with a disabled person and the perhaps awkwardness of our response, the scenes of dying children in a country ravaged by famine and civil war, the gradual deterioration of a friend through a debilitating and degenerative illness—all serve to act as events of irruption and intrusion into our lives, and force us to become sufferers who suffer for others. And the process of our suffering will follow the same path, and will throw up the same emotions and the same questions that bring about a sense of doubt in who we think we are.

Not all of us suffer in the same way; our personal histories and the relationships we share with other people ensure that the context of suffering is unique in its impact on a person's sense of identity. However, suffering is an unavoidable experience of personal life—not in the negative sense of being something we should or ought to avoid, but in the positive sense of being a presence in our lives which forges, either creatively or destructively, the sense of our own identity and the kind of person we wish to become. To suffer is to be a person; suffering lies at the heart of personal identity. This is not to say that suffering is therefore "necessary," or to be encouraged, or that those who do not suffer are any less a person than those who do (but I reject the claim any person does not suffer). The claim is that suffering, or the possibility of suffering, is an integral part of what it is to be a person. And alongside the recognition that suffering is an integral feature of personal experience must come the recognition that suffering—whether in us or in those around us—is therefore not an unwelcome "addition" to a person's life, it instead forms part of the foundations of a person's identity.

Persons, identity, and suffering are not three separable elements; they form a complex and constantly evolving package which denotes the nature of personal life on earth.

Two

WRITING THE DISASTER: INSCRIPTIONS OF THE SELF

H. Mike Awalt

> Gradually it has become clear to me what every great philosophy so far has been: namely, the personal confession of its author and a kind of involuntary and unconscious memoir. (Friedrich Nietzsche, *Beyond Good and Evil*)

This chapter is concerned with writing, with philosophy, with autobiography, and with the limits that give rise to all three and which in turn all three try to inscribe and transgress. Writing, philosophy, autobiography—the lines between them blur and they merge. All are attempts to inscribe the self and to write the disaster.

1.

What is disaster, and what does it mean to write the disaster? In our ordinary language, disaster means destructive violence in the case of natural events like the floods in southern California and the earthquakes in Japan, or it means the complete failure of projects or expectations. Webster's dictionary defines disaster as "any happening that causes great harm or damage; sudden misfortune; calamity."[1] For the purposes of this chapter, disaster is defined as those absurd events which shatter the continuities of our experiences and break the moral sense through which we understand and order our lives. Its presence undercuts the ways in which we maintain our security and wholeness. John Caputo examines the derivation of the term, stating that "to suffer disaster is to lose one's star (dis-astrum), to be cut loose from one's lucky or guiding light....Is that not what a disaster means? That the star-guide stories that take us by the hand through the storms and tempests of factical life have lost their credibility."[2]

The exact nature of the disaster is relative to the individual. It may be an intense inner awareness or a sweeping, destructive public event. Yet its effects are the same in that, as Paul Tillich says, we experience "the shaking of the foundations" that undergird us and become painfully aware of our own mortality and finitude. Søren Kierkegaard's experiences with his father and with Regine, and Elie Wiesel's experiences in Auschwitz fall under this definition of disaster. Though different experiences, they radically disrupt and unsettle the lives and projects of those who experienced them. Though one appears trivial in comparison with the horrific nature of the other, what is significant is the nature of the effect the event had on the individual who experienced it.

Though integrally connected with death, disaster is not personal demise, in that the self who experiences disaster is not eradicated but remains. Though touched by it, this self is spared. This sparing is part of the disaster. Maurice Blanchot in the opening lines of *The Writing of the Disaster*, underscores this fact:

> The disaster ruins everything, all the while leaving everything intact. It does not touch anyone in particular; 'I' am not threatened by it, but spared, left aside. It is in this way that I am threatened; it is in this way that the disaster threatens in me that which is exterior to me—an Other than I who passively becomes Other.[3]

The nature of disaster is predicated on and symbolized by a more fundamental philosophical awareness that a limit to human thought and action exists, an Other or outside that evades all human attempts to order, think, and domesticate it and which perpetually bankrupts all our attempts to systematize and unify our ways of being in the world. The notion of disaster points to that aspect of nature and experience which always disrupts our attempts to gain control and to infuse meaning and order into the flow and fragmentary quality of life. A direct relation appears between the success of our attempts to gain control through the thrust of modern technological society and the nature and severity of the disaster. The more we think we can banish disorder, the more shattering its lingering, recalcitrant presence.

Blanchot says that the disaster, though it evades our attempts in language to express it and evokes initially only silence from us, gives rise to writing. We must seek to write the disaster, even though that writing will always be fragmentary and incomplete. In no way can we totally name or inscribe the disaster. When all has been said, it still stands unexhausted and inexhaustible. "When all is said; what remains to be said is the disaster. Ruin of words, demise of writing, faintness faintly murmuring; what remains without remains (the fragmentary)."[4] In the closing lines of *The Writing of the Disaster*, Blanchot hauntingly states, "What remains to be said. Shining solitude, the void of the sky, a deferred death; disaster."[5] The book jacket to Blanchot's work has this penetrating account of his work and of the task of writing the disaster:

> How can we write or think about disaster when by its nature it defies speech or compels silence—when, moreover, it consumes thought and rips books apart? We cannot; but writing, Blanchot says, is the patient response of this helplessness. He reflects upon writing that attempts to

> abide in the disaster's infinite threat, attempts even to dwell in its fellowship, without thereby abandoning the other link, which is to describe, explain, prevent, redeem, or redefine the dread and pain. [6]

In the midst of a disaster which shatters the mask of order we have placed around our lives, which leaves us wounded but still standing, and in the face of the abyss which brings us face to face with those aspects of life that refuse to be neatly incorporated into any sensible narrative, we nonetheless must write. We must try to express what eludes expression.

2.

The case could be made that the writings of many philosophers—Augustine, Rousseau, Kierkegaard, Nietzsche, and Wittgenstein—constitute a writing of the disaster. I will focus on three attempts to write the disaster: Plato, Kierkegaard, and Wiesel.

The disaster that marks the life and work of Plato is the death of Socrates. The story of Socrates goes something like this. Socrates is a haunting figure who devoted his life to conversation. Much like Kierkegaard, over 2,200 years later, he wandered the streets of his community engaging the learned people of his day in dialogue. Driven by a desire for knowledge, a disdain for the pretenses of knowledge in his peers, and the awareness of his ignorance, Socrates roamed the community of Athens, relentlessly questioning and dismantling the views of others. With great zest, he attacked those who prided themselves in their knowledge and in their status in the city and uncovered the groundlessness of their views. Socrates's self-chosen role as gadfly to the community of Athens earned him the admiration of the young intellectuals and the wrath of the elders of the city. He was brought to trial on the charges of corrupting the youth and atheism and convicted to death. Plato was one of those who followed Socrates and saw in him the life of reason given full shape and form. For Plato, Socrates was the paradigm of goodness. If human beings and the community they constituted were to reach their full potential, it would be through the process of self-examination that Socrates initiated.

Given this perception of Socrates, coupled with the well-documented Greek pride in the superiority of their culture, way of life, and intelligence, we should not be surprised that the death of Socrates created extreme trauma for Plato. It was incomprehensible that the best of men could be condemned and executed by the best of societies. This paradoxical happening flew in the face of the reason so cherished by the Greeks. Socrates's death constituted a disaster for Plato of foundation shaking proportions. Though Plato mentions he was at the trial of Socrates, what is intriguing is that Plato mentions in the *Phaedo* (the dialogue which recreates the death of Socrates) that he was not present at the dialogue he is reporting. He is not present at the death of Socrates. According to tradition, Plato was too ill. Ascribing interior motives to personages over two millennia removed from us is risky; however, we can plausibly conjecture that Plato is debilitated by the prospect of Socrates's execution and can't bring himself to be present.

Socrates's fate made it no longer possible to view Athens or its government in the same way. Plato leaves Athens after the execution and commences a nomadic journey that takes him throughout the Mediterranean world and possibly as far away as Egypt. Twelve years later, he returns to Athens, and, though exact dates about the chronology of his writings are impossible, a case could be made that ten years elapse before he writes about the event. The initial response to the disaster is silence. We are mute. Only silence can do justice to the experience of devastation.

However, when Plato does begin to write, it is the disaster that must be written. *Euthypro*, *The Apology*, and *Crito* are recognized as Plato's earliest dialogues. They all center around the trial and imprisonment of Socrates. In *The Apology,* Plato gives Socrates's defense at his trial and artfully tries to answer the question, "Who is Socrates?" In the opening line of *The Apology*, Socrates says that his accusers are so adept and convincing that they almost made him forget who he was. In the discourse that follows through the three linked dialogues, one gets a portrait in the *logos* of Socrates.

Blanchot states that the disaster cannot be grasped and rendered in comprehensible language, and thus in any public terms. However, we can't get away from it. It haunts us, disrupting our "solitude and overflows every variety of thought, as the intense, silent, and disastrous affirmation of the outside."[7] Plato can't walk away from it. Most scholars divide Plato's work into three chronological periods; early, middle, and late. In the middle period, a good twenty years removed from the event, the disaster is still present in the middle of his writing and in the middle of his masterpiece, *The Republic*, disrupting the attempts to construct in words and thought the perfect city and to found justice in the world.

In the "Parable of the Cave," Plato depicts an underground world in which human beings are chained in such a way that they believe a world of shadows is the real world. They are comfortable in this world of darkness and have adapted to it. One day, one of the prisoners is released. For the first time, he sees the world of the cave from a new perspective. He ascends out of the darkness of the cave and into the world of light and truth. This is where we would like to end this parable. The assent out of darkness into light is slow, sure, but permanent. Once we get there, we never have to return to darkness. This reading would parallel Plato's, "Divided Line" that is told at the end of Book VI of *The Republic*. In that story, reality is divided into two levels—the transitory world of ordinary experience and the world of forms (the real world). Each of the two parts of the line have two areas. A type of thinking is related to each object of knowledge. The message of the story is that human reason can move from the lower forms of knowledge to the higher forms in unhindered fashion, and certain knowledge can be attained through the exercise of reason while we are still in this world.

Plato's Cave parable does not end here. The prisoner is taken back down into the cave where he must adjust to the world of darkness. But now he knows the difference between illusion and reality, and he proceeds to tell the prisoners of their plight and of the wonderful world that lies outside the cave. The prisoners, however, think he has lost his mind and would kill him if they could get the opportunity. This story falls in the midst of a long book about justice and the search for a perfect society. Earlier in *The Republic*, we have been told that in order for a perfect society to exist, the philosopher—that is, the one who knows, who has seen the real world and has encountered genuine knowledge—must rule. However, the paradox is that what is necessary is what society cannot tolerate—the philosopher. The story is a thinly disguised reference to Socrates. In this attempt to bring justice into the world, the disaster rears its head again and interrupts all attempts at completeness and order. The reality of Socrates's death won't go away and must be written again and again. Blanchot says:

> In Plato's cave, there is no word to designate death, and no dream or image to intimate its unspeakableness. Death is there, in the cave, as excess, and forgetfully; it arrives from outside into the words of the philosopher as that which reduces him in advance to silence.[8]

The disaster still stands, unrelieved and unincorporated; a fragmentary tear in the rational fabric of reality which can't be stated and yet paradoxically must be written.

Jacques Derrida, in *The Ear of the Other*, states that the autobiography is the telling of my life to myself. This telling originates from a principle of contradiction—death (father) and life (mother). The autobiographical signature is written in the singular step between life and death. "It remains a line of credit opened onto eternity and refers back to one of the two I's, the nameless parties of the contract."[9] Though writing about Nietzsche, Derrida's comments appear relevant here. Plato's writing issues from these two contradictions—life (the power of Socrates's questioning and reasoning) and death (the Athenian execution of Socrates). These two forces give rise to Plato's early work.

3.

The disaster that marks Kierkegaard's life is more complex and difficult to pinpoint. We might more appropriately say disasters. Kierkegaard's life was marked by a series of crises, some of which were forced by Kierkegaard himself. His writing seemed to flow out of conflicts—the intellectual conflict with Hegel and the Danish Hegelians, the battle with the newspaper, *The Corsair*, and the struggle with the Danish Lutheran Church. All of these were public encounters in which Kierkegaard usually came out as the villain. However, two relationships proved to be the most shattering for Kierkegaard and constitute the disasters he found it necessary to write.

Kierkegaard, a self-styled poet and "witness to the truth," produced a voluminous amount of written work between 1843 and his death in 1855. In addition to over 15 published works, he kept a journal of assorted papers and letters (20 volumes in the Danish edition). Much of this material mirrors his life. The membrane between his life and his work is thin.

Kierkegaard was born in 1813, when his father, Michael Pedersen Kierkegaard was fifty-seven years of age. Søren, the youngest of seven children, was raised in an atmosphere of extreme religious devotion and discipline. On more than one occasion in his journals, he talks of never having experienced childhood, and of coming into the world an old man. "Why did I not thrive as other children do, why was I not wrapped around in joy, why did I come into that region of sighs so early... so that I was not born like other children but was born old."[10]

Søren is not responsible for his "being born old." He inherited it and his pervasive sense of guilt from his father, who was obsessed with acts out of his past. Michael Pedersen Kierkegaard grew up in poverty on the Jutland Heath. One day while tending sheep in the isolated cold of this barren region, he raised his fist to the heavens and cursed God. Shortly thereafter, Michael Pedersen's fortunes changed for the better. He was sent to work for his uncle in Copenhagen. He worked hard, developed a subsidiary business, and eventually inherited his uncle's estate. Every venture he tried in the realm of business was a success. His wealth grew, but so did his melancholy and his guilt. Michael Pedersen could not forget that cold, distant (but yet so near), day on the Jutland Heath, and was convinced that judgment was imminent. He came to believe that the curse would be exercised on his family and that his wealth was a part of his penalty. He would be condemned to outlive all of his children and so his wealth would come to nothing.

He conveyed this mood of melancholy, guilt, and impending demise to all of his children. With this sense of doom hanging heavy over his head, he retired from business the year Søren was born and dedicated himself to raising Søren for the service of God. One night, years later, a young Søren Kierkegaard overheard his penitent father fervently confessing a terrible sin. Although Søren doesn't state the nature of his discovery, he tells a story in *Stages on Life's Way* entitled "Solomon's dream" in which a young Solomon overhears his father (King David) confessing his sin with Bathsheba. Most scholars feel that the story is transparent and is a thinly veiled telling of his shattering discovery of his father's indiscretion. The secret he learns about his father further complicates an already ambivalent relationship.

In his journals, Søren says, "Merciful God, what a dreadful wrong my father did me in his melancholy—an old man who unloads all his depression on a poor child, to say nothing of what was even more dreadful, and yet for all that the best of fathers."[11] The dead father, as Derrida says, is already absent to himself, leaving the son a legacy of guilt and death. The father inscribes his melancholy on the persona of the son—Kierkegaard. In Danish, the word means churchyard or cemetery.

The other side of the tension between death/life appears strangely missing. In Kierkegaard's writing, his mother is absent, except for one cryptic comment in the journals: "Children who remember their mother."[12] Though references to the father abound, the mother is nowhere to be found—even on the date of her death (1834, four years before the death of Søren's father). Nothing feminine is alive here.

But Regine Olson is present. Søren and Regine met at her house in 1837. She was 14, and he was 23. In September 1840, they were engaged. According to Kierkegaard's journals, he regretted his decision immediately. "The next day I saw that I had made a mistake. Penitent that I was, ... my melancholy, that was sufficient."[13]

The break with Regine was immediately followed by intense literary production. After the break-up, Søren left for Berlin where he attended Schelling's lectures on philosophy and started work on *Either/Or*, which he claims he wrote in just eleven months. He returned to Copenhagen where he published *Either/Or* in 1843. One day at church, he spotted Regine, and she nodded at him—twice—and according to Kierkegaard, "looked at him fervently." Within a few weeks, Kierkegaard fled Copenhagen again for the security of "distant" Berlin, and wrote. He brought *Repetition* and *Fear and Trembling* from pen to press before the end of the year.

The presence (or is it absence?) of Regine dominates his journal entries. As late as 1852, frequent reflections still appear on her, his sacrifice in giving her up, and the possibility of reestablishing the relationship (a doubtful prospect since she had married in 1848).

Scholars have speculated that Kierkegaard did not marry Regine because he feared that he lived under a family curse and did not want to bring any more descendants into that lineage of extreme melancholy. Though he did not marry and did not sire any children, Søren sired a minimum of four literary offspring (all pseudonymous and thus illegitimate) as a result of the intellectual conjoining with Regine. In an entry dated in 1848, he says, "as soon as I die (which I continually expect to happen soon), she of course will be reinstated in her rights. Everything is ready for that. Her name will belong to my authorship and be remembered as long as I am remembered."[14] In another entry, dated a year later, he says, "she was the beloved. My life will unconditionally accent her life, my literary work is to be regarded as a monument to her honor and praise. I take her along into history."[15] Regarding her as the idealized wife she was, he left her his work (including the journals and papers) and bequeathed his estate, now spent except for his words, to his "own dear little Regine."

The dead father and the living feminine, the accounts out of which he opens his line of credit, are principles of contradiction through which the name, Søren Kierkegaard, arises:

> If I were asked how, apart from my relationship to God, I was disciplined to be an author, I would answer: By an old man, to whom I am most grateful, and a young girl, to whom I am most indebted—to that unity of age and youth, of the severity of winter and the gentleness of summer which must also have been a natural potentiality within me; the former disciplined me with his noble wisdom, the other with her loving unwisdom. [16]

In another journal entry, Kierkegaard states that "I came to understand myself by writing."[17] He was driven to write the disaster to try to understand these shattering events, and, in so doing, to understand himself.

One example will suffice. In *Fear and Trembling*, Kierkegaard deals with the biblical story of Abraham and Isaac. The book tries to make sense of Abraham's willingness to sacrifice Isaac. How could a father surrender his son in response to a perceived command of God? We can easily see the work as Kierkegaard's struggle with his relationship with his father. His father is Abraham, while he is Isaac. Søren has been sacrificed by his father and has been condemned to a life of melancholy. Yet we can turn this story another way. At one and the same time, it reflects Søren's relationship with Regine. Søren is Abraham, while Regine is Isaac. He has sacrificed her for religious reasons. *Fear and Trembling* is Kierkegaard's attempt to write his disaster. He says in a journal entry that "he who understands *Fear and Trembling*, understands the riddle of my life." However, he cannot fully comprehend what has happened. He must write, but the writing always fails to fully inscribe the disaster or the self who survives it. In *Fear and Trembling*, Johannes de Silentio, the philosophical poet who is trying to tell Abraham's story, finally says that He stands there in silence. He cannot understand Abraham. He can only be his poet.

The paradoxical problem of needing to tell his story and being unable to tell it, propels Kierkegaard's autobiographical discourse. The need and drive to understand himself is a necessary one. Kierkegaard says that "in frightful inner suffering I became an author."[18] Kierkegaard's sense of disaster arising from the relationships which marked his life (his father, Regine, the affair with *The Corsair*, and the church) compelled him to write. According to Blanchot, Kierkegaard has to thematize the secret to deal with the suffering that arises from his need to tell all and his inability to tell all. Communication occurs only when what is written becomes the sign of what is hidden.

Kierkegaard has to write. He has to try to understand himself. He must tell the secret that haunts him. He must explain his unique individuality in public terms. This is a necessity. He cannot put it down or step away from it. He wants to quit, but discovers that he cannot.

Repeatedly in his journals, Kierkegaard's contradictory, shifting discourse reveals the ambiguity he experiences in his effort to penetrate to the core of himself. He admits to the tension he experiences as he tries to adhere to the Socratic dictum to know himself. He says that from the beginning he has been in contradiction to himself, but he affirms that a person's true self will come through this opposition. Later, in that same entry, what appears resolved begins to unravel as the discourse continues:

> When a judge is uncertain, he conducts an interrogation, pursues every clue, and then pronounces a judgment—that is, he comes to the conclusion: guilty or innocent; but now and then he dismisses the charge. Is then nothing accomplished by that judgment? Indeed there is—the uncertainty is determined. He was uncertain as to how he should judge; now he is no longer uncertain, now his verdict is ready: he judges that he is uncertain. He rests in that, for one cannot rest in uncertainty, but one can rest when one has determined it. [19]

The movement of the discourse points toward the uncertainty that lies at the heart of Søren Kierkegaard, an uncertainty he has determined:

> The lake is not easy to approach, for it is surrounded by a rather wide stretch of quagmire. Here the boundary dispute between the lake and the land goes on night and day. There is something melancholy about this battle, of which, however no trace of destruction gives any indication, for what the earth wins from the lake is transformed into a smiling and exceedingly fertile meadow. Ah, but the poor lake that is disappearing in this way. [20]

The necessity and the impossibility of the struggle to know the self continues throughout human existence. On the surface no damage appears. In Kierkegaard's case, he has his literary work, the smiling meadow produced out of the boundary dispute between lake and land. But the lake is disappearing, death approaches and he is no closer to answering the question of what it means to be Søren Kierkegaard. He says:

> but then I cannot, after all, say: I. At most I can say (that is, given my scrupulous demand for the truth): this is how I now understand the productivity of the past. The flaw, again, is that if I do not do it myself, there is no one who can present it, for no one knows it the way I do. No

> one can explain the structure of the whole as I can. But this is my limitation—I am a pseudonym. Fervently, incitingly, I present the ideal, and when the listener or reader is moved to tears, then I still have one job left: to say, "I am not that, my life is not like that." Quite true: I feel I would be able to be more effective if at this moment someone stepped forward and spoke in his name and gesticulated with his life. [21]

Kierkegaard affirmed a private mystery in every soul that could not become public. Sylviane Agacinski states, "The secret is unpublishable because it has no language, not even for the one it constitutes and holds in secret, from himself."[22]

Though Blanchot talks about the disaster in general terms, the one event in the twentieth century that is marked by that term and which stands as the paradigmatic case, is the Holocaust.

4.

For Blanchot, the Holocaust is the disaster. He states:

> The unknown name, alien to naming: The holocaust, the absolute event of history—which is a date in history—that utter-burn where all history took fire, where the movement of Meaning was swallowed up, there the gift, which knows nothing of forgiving or, consent, shattered without giving place to anything that can be affirmed, that can be denied—gift of passivity, gift of what cannot be given. How can it be preserved, even by thought? How can thought be made the keeper of the holocaust where all was lost, including guardian thought? In the mortal intensity, the fleeing silence of the countless crying. [23]

The Holocaust haunts Elie Wiesel. As a deeply religious 15-year-old, he was, along with his family and his community of Sighet, Romania, loaded into cattle cars and shipped to a concentration camp. Over the next year or so, he spent time in Auschwitz, Buna, and Buchenwald. He witnessed the death of his mother, father, and sister, as well as the God of his youth. He writes in *Night*:

> Never shall I forget that night, the first night in camp, which has turned my life into one long night, seven times cursed and seven times sealed. Never shall I forget that smoke. Never shall I forget the little faces of the children whose bodies I saw turned into wreaths of smoke beneath a silent blue sky.
>
> Never shall I forget those flames which consumed my faith forever. Never shall I forget that nocturnal silence which deprived me, for all eternity, of

> the desire to live. Never shall I forget those moments which murdered my God and my soul and turned my dreams to dust. Never shall I forget these things, even if I am condemned to live as long as God himself. Never. [24]

After he was released from Buchenwald in 1945, Wiesel was, in his words, a corpse. He recalls looking at himself in a mirror in a hospital: "From the depths of the mirror, a corpse gazed back at me. The look in his eyes, as they stared into mine, has never left me."[25]

For ten years, he lived under a self-imposed silence, choosing not to violate the memory of that event by trying to express it in words. When the disaster allowed itself to be written, it poured forth, 860 pages in the Yiddish version. Yet, Wiesel could not let it all be said. Some things must remain unsayable, some secrets must never be told. When he rewrote it in French, it was 109 pages. Wiesel believes that some things cannot be said. The disaster must be written, but it cannot all be written. In 1993, Oprah Winfrey asked him to tell about the last time he saw his mother and his sister. Nearly fifty years after the night he witnessed their death, it could not be said. He shook his head and was silent. Blanchot says that "it is not you who will speak, let the disaster speak in you, even if it be by your forgetfulness or silence."[26] Through his silence, the disaster was spoken, inscribed in our minds by the eloquence of his silence.

Numerous times in this chapter, I have spoken of the inability of language to express the disaster—of the disaster lying outside of thought and expression. In Wiesel's interview with Winfrey, this point surfaces repeatedly. In one exchange, Oprah said, "I read *Night*, but I can't conceive of it." Wiesel says, "you can't conceive of it, no words are strong enough to convey it, no matter how good the writer is. The tale is so grotesque that it must be the tale of a madman. Sanity and reason could not tell such a tale. How could something like this happen in civilized Europe and the whole world remain silent?"

In writing the disaster, Wiesel enables us to draw near and be moved by that experience that we cannot even think. In the preface to the Bantam edition of *Night*, Robert McAfee Brown states:

> The rest of us, who have not inhabited the inner most circle of hell, can never know what it was like to be there. But between us and the fiery furnaces where they burned babies alive stands the presence of Elie Wiesel, his presence casts a shadow from within which we can see, in dimmest outline, the reality he saw and touched and tasted directly. [27]

Brown states, "he tells the story, out of infinite pain, partly to honor the dead, but also to warn the living that it could happen again and that it must never happen again. Better that one heart be broken a thousand times in the retelling, he has decided, it means that a thousand other hearts need not be broken at all."[28]

Writing the disaster. The claim of this chapter has been that the philosophical and literary works of these three men constitutes their attempt to inscribe the disaster that marks their lives. Though radically different in nature and severity, in each case the disaster served to break the moral continuity and order of life and to shake the foundations that give life meaning and sense. This tear in the fabric of life in each case does not fade with the passing of time, but stays vivid and unmendable. As Wiesel says, the more time passes, the stronger the memories become and the more he remembers. The nature of the disaster is that it doesn't go away.

The writing of disaster does not enable us to understand fully the catastrophe or to set it aside and move to something else. Plato can not get away from the disaster. Years later, he is still grappling with it and the power of the disaster is still giving birth to literary pieces. This is especially true in the cases of writers like Kierkegaard and Wiesel, where we can plausibly argue that everything they have written is the writing of the disaster. They must perpetually write, not to get it right, but to inscribe what is always fragmentary. Writing does not heal the self or redeem the self. On the contrary, writing keeps the wound open and keeps us aware of the impossibility or undesirability of completely closing the circle.

Yet, in that wound, that fissure, and in the attempt to inscribe it, light, meaning, truth, and discovery, appear. Though the darkness remains, light occurs. In Plato's cave, darkness is still there, but so is light. The light is Plato's writing which keeps Socrates and his questions alive.

In his discussion of disaster, Caputo maintains that the disaster is an economic notion. When one suffers a disaster, one suffers irretrievable loss. No return balances the books and offsets the loss. Excessive spending without return marks the disaster. Caputo says, "by irretrievable loss I mean a wasting of life, something that cannot be repaired, recompensated, redeemed. A disaster is a loss that cannot be incorporated into a 'result,' that cannot be led back into a gain."[29]

Though I agree with Caputo's notion of no return and would agree that nothing can be brought forth to offset the negativity of disaster, something does issue from the disaster—the writing. Though it does not explain, justify, or redeem the event, such writing is there as a work wrought in response to the event.

Blanchot says, "It is dark disaster that brings light."[30] The light that is brought is the body of work produced. Dark disaster is the well spring of the creativity that produces the masterpieces of writers like Plato, Kierkegaard, and Wiesel. Their writing is the light that enlightens the reader. They don't negate the darkness, but they stand defiantly against it, casting their flickering light in its midst.

5.

To hear Blanchot, Plato, Kierkegaard, and Wiesel, is to begin to think philosophy in a new way. The history of Western philosophy has been predominantly the story of the attempt to fill in the gaps and to create a view of the world that ties everything together with reason. It strives to provide an overarching vision in which everything makes sense if we work hard enough. Ironically, the Western tradition claims Plato as its originary voice. This chapter counters with the possibility that philosophy's fundamental purpose is not to bring closure. It must resist that basic desire and must strive to give voice to what is unthinkable and unsayable. Philosophy must give voice to those fragments that can never fit into any system. It must not cover this voice over and try to incorporate it into some artificial system of meaning, so that the voice is lost. Philosophy must tarry with it and seek to write it and by so writing, let it speak. As Blanchot says, the disaster is a gift of terror and possibility. Plato, in keeping Socrates alive, keeps alive terror and possibility.

Not only does writing the disaster force us to leave the wound open, therefore seeing philosophy in a new light, it also forces us to understand ourselves in a new light. The disaster gives shape to who we are. It does not destroy us, but it inscribes us. Selves are constructed, not given. Out of the struggle with the disaster and the attempt to give it a voice, we, in the process, shape our own voice. Plato and Kierkegaard have inscripted themselves in the act of writing the disaster. Since the wound is forever open, the self is forever in the process of being inscribed. To close the wound is to close the wellspring out of which the self grows.

To summarize, I close this chapter with a quotation from Blanchot. He says:

> Granted, Socrates does not write, but beneath the voice, it is nevertheless through writing that he gives himself to others as the perpetual subject perpetually destined to die. He does not speak, he questions. Questioning, he interrupts and interrupts himself without cease, giving form ironically to the fragmentary; through his death (the disaster) he causes speech to be haunted by writing, and therein limits writing to a single form: that of the testament....[31]

NOTES

1. *Webster's II: New Riverside Dictionary* (New York: Berkley Books, 1984), p. 200.

2. John Caputo, *Against Ethics* (Bloomington, Ind.: Indiana University Press, 1993), p. 6.

3. Maurice Blanchot, *The Writing of the Disaster*, trans. Ann Smock (Lincoln, Neb.: University of Nebraska Press, 1986), p. 1.

4. *Ibid.*, p. 33.

5. *Ibid.*, p. 146.

6. *Ibid.*, book jacket.

7. *Ibid.*, p. 5.

8. *Ibid.*, p. 35.

9. Jacques Derrida, *The Ear of the Other*, trans. Peggy Kamuf (Lincoln, Neb.: University of Nebraska Press, 1985), p. 16.

10. *Søren Kierkegaard's Journals and Papers*, ed. and trans. H.V. Hong and E. Hong (7 vols.; Bloomington, Indiana: Indiana University Press, 1967-1978), Vol. 5, pp. 232-233.

11. *Ibid.*, 6, p. 202.

12. *Ibid.*, 5, p. 70.

13. *Ibid.*, 5, p. 193.

14. *Ibid.*, 6, p. 202.

15. *Ibid.*, 6, p. 55.

16. *Ibid.*, 6, p. 158.

17. *Ibid.*, 6, p. 37.

18. *Ibid.*, 6, p. 444.

19. *Ibid.*, 5, p. 219.

20. Søren Kierkegaard, *Stages on Life's Way*, trans. and ed. H. V. Hong and E. Hong (Princeton: Princeton University Press, 1988), p. 187.

21. *Ibid.*, 6, pp. 231-232.

22. Sylviane Agacinski, *Aparte: Conceptions and Deaths of Søren Kierkegaard*, trans. Kevin Newmark (Tallahassee: Florida State University Press, 1988), p. 190.

23. Blanchot, *The Writing of the Disaster*, p. 46.

24. Elie Wiesel, *Night*, trans. S. Rodway (New York: Bantam Books, 1960), p. 32.

25. *Ibid.*, p. 109.

26. Blanchot, *The Writing of the Disaster*, p. 4.

27. Robert McAfee Brown, "Preface for the Twenty-Fifth Anniversary Edition" in Wiesel, *Night*, p. vi.

28. *Ibid.*, p. v.

29. Caputo, *Against Ethics*, p. 27.

30. Blanchot, *The Writing of the Disaster*, p. 7.

31. *Ibid.*, p. 65.

Three

THE CRY FOR HUMAN WORTH

David A. Pailin

In July 1994, I visited a British War Cemetery in North Africa. As I wandered around the carefully tended lines of tombstones, I wondered who these people were. Many had names on them, but who now remembered them? Some were marked "Known only to God." Who had they been? And then I thought about the bodies that were left in the streets in Rwanda, the heaps of skulls in Cambodia—Kampuchea, the mass graves of the German concentration camps. And so one could go on. History may preserve the stories of some world–historical figures but for the huge majority of human beings, the passage of time is a journey into the void. What may realistically be claimed about the worth of human beings?

As John Macquarrie points out, "a human being is, in essence, constituted by a contradiction or even a conflict." While, the "unalterable fact of finitude...must be taken into account in any realistic description of what it means to exist in the human condition," human beings are "constituted by a wide range of possibilities and capacities" that challenge them, as self–conscious living beings, continually to reach out beyond their present bounds. "Weak and hemmed in as each one of us may be, there is in us (call it by the traditional name of spirit) that leaps out into the infinite realm of being surrounding us."[1] Nevertheless, however strong a call to venture towards the novel and the infinite may characterize human existence, claims about the significance and worth of human being, whether considered corporately or individually, are faced by fundamental threats. [2]

Human existence is a minute episode in the cosmological story of an undistinguished star system in a physically unremarkable galaxy. Biological understanding of the chance and necessity mode of evolution of DNA macro-molecules render implausible traditional—and still widespread—descriptions of the nature of human being as the intentional implementation of divine designs. The basic genetic structure of any individual is the point of a cone of largely accidental interactions whose number doubles with each generation back. Historical records report the existence and sometimes parts of the story of some persons but of most people that have lived no records exist: "there are others who are unremembered; they are dead, and it is as though...they had never been born" (Ecclesiasticus 44:9). The social dimensions of human existence mean that, apart from a few rare individuals, most people for most of the time are puppets in mass movements of whose dynamics they have little awareness and over which they have even less control. In the past century studies of human personality, developing the pioneering investigations of Freud and Jung, have indicated how subtle and often subconscious factors mold individual personality. Far from being the masters of their fate, human beings seem at times not to be the masters of their own decisions. Finally, as people grow older they find that even their own past disappears into oblivion. When I scan old diaries, I cannot recall many of the appointments that they list nor identify the persons that I was to meet. Individuals find that even their own past is largely lost for them.

This being so, what sense can be made of claims about the significance and worth of human beings? One theistic response that is arguably both credible and substantial is that presented by the notion of objective immortality (the doctrine that whereas the consciousness, experiences, and agency of a self are to be considered to end at the death of that self, the occasions that constituted that self are held to be everlastingly remembered—and so preserved as "objects"—in the consciousness of the divine). In the closing section of *Process and Reality*, for example, A. N. Whitehead maintains that "each actual entity in the temporal world" is received "into God's nature" where it is transmuted "into a temporal ever–present fact." "What is done in the world is transformed into a reality in heaven." What this means is that while each occasion—each droplet of experience that constitutes existence, however trivial—perishes in this world, it is "everlasting in the Being of God." Accordingly, on the grounds that God is to be understood in part as "the great companion—the fellow-sufferer who understands," Whitehead maintains that the insistent craving of our zest for existence is satisfied by the recognition that "our immediate actions" have "ever-present, unfading importance" since while in our experience of the processes of reality they perish once they have come to concrescence, in the reality of the divine they continue to "live for evermore" and contribute to God's continuing response to all future possibilities.[3]

According to the doctrine of objective immortality, that is, each experience, however slight, has two subjects: one is immediately felt by God, the other by the self that is the non-divine subject of the experience. In consequence, whereas for the non-divine self the moment of experience then perishes and memory of it increasingly fades away, as incorporated into the divine it is preserved with the vividness of its original immediacy. Further, in response to the suggestion that such preservation is not significant since the incorporation of each droplet of experience into the divine reality is comparable to adding a drop of rain to the oceans, it may be held that the divine awareness is a cherishing awareness that identifies, respects the integrity of, and cares for each item of "individual self-realization."[4]

Although the metaphysical and theistic basis of Whitehead's notion of objective immortality may be—and is—open to dispute, the notion itself may be held to satisfy traditional theistic notions of the significance of human actions that are more widely expressed mythologically in stories about a final judgement and what Richard Niebuhr alleges to be the basic and inescapably human conviction "that life is worth living" and that "individuals have intrinsic worth"[5]—or what Schubert Ogden describes as human beings' "ultimate confidence" in "the unconditioned meaningfulness" of their lives since "the world is finally meaningful and...our striving to realize values is not simply vain."[6]

This way of understanding the worth and significance of humans may also be held to satisfy doctrines that interpret the claim that humankind is to be understood as *in imago Dei* in terms of being *homo liber*, a self-conscious as well as conscious agency whose nature and destiny is to a crucial extent self-determinative. G. W. F. Hegel, for instance, puts it that "human freedom is the ultimate pivot upon which humanity turns,"[7] while Jean-Paul Sartre expresses the fundamental existentialist claim, both theistic and atheistic, as the belief that "existence comes before essence—or, if you will, that we must begin from the subjective."[8] As Peter Hodgson points out, this not only requires that human beings develop a concept of freedom that replaces "hierarchy by equality and dominion by reciprocity and mutual responsibility": it also entails the recognition that "human beings are free primarily by virtue of their capability to speak" for "language is the road to freedom...human being is 'created' when language emerges and the determinacy of nature gives way to the freedom of spirit."[9] Finally, as will be amplified later, the doctrine of objective immortality may be held to provide a way of understanding the significance and worth of human beings that fits the kind of insight into the mutual character of human beings that is put forward, for instance, by John Macmurray. By extending to the divine, the perception that the value of persons does not lie in their solitary individuality but in their relationships with others, it suggests that in some non-trivial respects the divine as the universal individual both gives and finds value through relationships with all others in ways that are most appropriate to each of those others.

Those who consider that the human craving for significance and worth is satisfied by the doctrine of objective immortality should, however, avoid thinking of human being in general and of individuals in particular more highly than is warrantable. Whitehead himself warned against such *hubris*. In a short piece on John Dewey, for example, he writes that:

> The human race consists of a small group of animals which for a small time has barely differentiated itself from the mass of animal life on a small planet circling round a small sun. The Universe is vast. Nothing is more curious than the self-satisfied dogmatism with which mankind at each period of its history cherishes the delusion of the finality of its existing modes of knowledge.[10]

However, proper humility does not entail worthlessness and insignificance. The doctrine that God, as absolutely loving, embraces and preserves every experience means that each and every human achievement is appreciated and, as such, forever contributes its proper value to the universal reality of the divine.

Attempts to establish such a doctrine, and other similar attempts by philosophers and theologians to warrant claims about the deep significance and worth of human beings, are always in danger of overlooking a problem that threatens their basic plausibility. This threat becomes apparent when we acknowledge that most discussions that concern the significance and worth of a human being also consider that human being primarily (and often—although unconsciously—definitively) in terms of the mode of existence that is possible for, if not experienced by, people who are in vital respects self-aware, responsible, and free. To a large extent the value of human beings is accordingly considered in terms of the possibilities open to those who are fairly affluent, educated, and able to make meaningful decisions about their existence. Human beings are thus understood by reference to the character and self-understanding of the middle classes of the First World and of those who belong to what are now denigrated as the "chattering classes" of the academic world—those, that is, who have time to think about their significance and the leisure to get worried about it. The concerns and experiences of such people (and I expect that those who read this chapter, like the writer, belong to this group) may not be typical of human beings and accordingly are not a sound basis for trying to make sense of the significance and worth of that being.

As I indicate in *A Gentle Touch: From a Theology of Handicap to a Theology of Human Being*, awareness of this point came to me through reflecting on the life of Alex.[11] In his early days Alex, who had Down's Syndrome, was so small that his mother borrowed a doll's cardigan from his sister for him to wear. He suffered from severe jaundice, problems with bone formation that led to spontaneous fractures, and an inguinal hernia. He had a one centimeter hole between the atria and severe pulmonary hypertension. He was eventually diagnosed as having Hirschsprung's Disease, a condition in which no nerves are present in the lower part of the bowel and which leads to constipation, distension, and extreme discomfort. Alex also learnt to smile, blow bubbles, and shake hands. Once he managed to sit unaided. He died when he was thirteen months old.[12]

For all the happy moments in his life and the "special magic" with which he elicited love in others, Alex's life challenges the view that the significance and worth of human beings is to be found in the preservation of their experiences and achievements in the divine reality. Whatever might be the case with a Socrates or a Siddhartha, a Genghis Khan or a Mozart, such a doctrine does not seem to establish much, if any, value for a life like that of Alex. What is hard to see, furthermore, is how Alex's life satisfies the anthropological analysis developed by Hodgson—an analysis, that is, that sees the human in terms of being *homo sapiens* and *homo liber*, rational, free and morally responsible, tragically sinful but also redeemable.[13] Or, to take another example, it does not seem to make a great deal of sense to try to apply to cases like that of Alex the view that the basic worth of human beings stems from being not only "a creature imbedded in the natural order," endowed with "physical and social impulses," but also a creature having "the freedom of his spirit," including both "transcendence over natural process" and "self–transcendence" that finds its true "source, end, and norm in the will of God" and through which a person "is able both to sin and to have some knowledge of his sin."[14]

While these questions were raised for me by reflecting on Alex's life, and my attempts to find some credible answers are offered in *A Gentle Touch*, it would be a mistake to consider that Alex's own existence poses the problem of human significance and worth in its most extreme form. This is not the case. As a friend pointed out to me after visiting a hospice for those who are in permanent severely disabled states, a credible (and so universally applicable) answer to the questions of human significance and worth must deal with more disturbing cases than that of Alex.

Alex, for instance, was aware to some degree of others and had some ability to respond—he returned smiles, blew bubbles, learned to shake hands, and eventually seemed to become worried at the sight of people in white coats. The media have recently drawn attention to the condition of a child who, while having some limited brain activity, is blind and deaf, has a fatal heart condition, can only be fed through a tube passed into his stomach, and whose behavior indicates that he is in constant pain. A recent news report stated that the doctors caring for this child were opposed to his parents' wish that he be allowed to die in a peaceful manner. The report made me wonder what is the criterion for "caring" in such circumstances. I am not convinced that to care for a person means in every case to seek to keep that person alive, whatever the costs to that person. Some people, however, have even more limited awareness; they seem to be largely unaware of their surroundings and unresponsive to stimuli.

Secondly, Alex was cherished by his parents, siblings, family, and friends. He received devoted care from them and from the medical staff who came into contact with him. This is not the situation of all people. Consideration of the significance of the human must take account of those for whom no one apparently cares—the neo-natal infant whose body is found wrapped in newspaper in a dustbin, the street child who lives in a sewer and is regarded as disposable by local traders, and the nameless old man whose corpse is found in a doorway.

Thirdly, although at times Alex writhed in discomfort and struggled for breath, much of the time he was a happy child who seemed contented and comfortable. Comprehensive accounts of the human condition, however, must include consideration of those whose waking existence is persistently and unrelievably racked by severe discomfort. People exist for whom every movement arouses physical pain and others whose state is such that they exist in continuous states of mental misery.

Fourthly, while Alex suffered from Down's Syndrome and died before he could develop many social skills, he appeared comfortable with himself and among people. He did not seem to suffer from the waking terrors and sleeping nightmares nor from the psychological disruptions and emotional disturbances that blight the existence of some people.

Finally, any credible understanding of the significance and worth of human beings must take account of the great numbers of humankind for whom existence does not appear to be a series of opportunities for value-creating achievements but a pointless, wearisome meandering to be endured. They are not heroic strugglers for survival but people who have not yet happened to die. As they trudge through unrewarding drudgeries, they may well empathize with the gravestone written by a domestic servant that is reported to read:

> Don't weep for me now,
> Don't weep for me ever,
> For I'm not going to work for never and never.

Whatever, then, may be affirmed about the nature of the person and about the significance and worth of human beings needs to account for all members of humankind. An interpretation of the human that is restricted to only one part of humankind—and that an economically and educationally privileged part—is worryingly defective. That discussions of the nature and value of persons must apply to all persons was an insight that came to me through Alex.

But if this is accepted, what may be affirmed about the significance and worth of human beings? Some suggested answers to this question appear on examination to be unsatisfactory.

One response holds that the question as it has been outlined above is *mal posé* and that properly understood the problem raised by the state of the disabled is far from novel. The justification claimed for this response is that the issue of disability is not to be tackled as part of anthropological understanding but as one aspect of the problem of natural evil. Disability, therefore, is an aspect of a problem that has confronted theists ever since religious belief developed the notion of God as the creator and sustainer of all that is and that has become acute wherever theists further hold that God is benevolent and wise as well as supremely powerful. Granted these beliefs, questions arise as to why the divine has either produced or permitted to be produced states of affairs—natural conditions, diseases, disabilities, and so on—that seem contrary to the divine will.

According to this response, then, the states of disabled people do pose a problem for theistic belief. But this problem does not concern the significance and worth of human beings. It concerns the existence of what are deemed to be states of natural evil in the created order. The question of human significance and worth is to be investigated in terms of the states and opportunities of the non-disabled.

This response, nevertheless, is flawed in numerous respects. In the first place, it fails to recognize adequately that reflection on the state of the disabled does not identify them as exceptions to the human condition but suggests that their state highlights the finite, limited state of all human beings. If this suggestion is followed up, as arguably it ought to be, the disabled are not to be regarded as exceptions to the human state but as vital reminders of the *hubris* with which attempts to tackle the question of the significance and worth of human beings often fail to appreciate the radically creaturely status of the human.

Secondly, this response suggests that since somewhere (in the Creator's design, for instance) an ideal pattern for human beings exists, a problem arises when some are found not to satisfy the requirements of that standard. But no evidence suggests that such a standard even exists, let alone what it may be. Any such notion is in any case deeply suspect biologically. The most adequate model of human beings currently available sees them as products of an evolutionary natural order whose genetic mutations seem to be due to occasional failures in the replication of macromolecules and to the consequences of accidental collisions of particles. The notion of a standard pattern for human beings is also suspect anthropologically, socially, and politically since those who are tempted to maintain that such a standard does exist seem to be in danger of adopting a master-race ideology that writes off those who do not satisfy the standard within designated limits—limits which presumably they themselves have determined since no objective standard to which reference can be made exists. They are thereby liable to be seeking, in effect, to deify their own state for what is unlikely in that any adopting this position would consciously adopt a standard that excluded themselves.

Thirdly, and fundamentally, this response fails to appreciate that while the problem of evil does point to some aspects of what the issue of human worth may involve theistically, it is itself arguably a problem that is, at the present time, *mal posé*. This is because it does not seem possible at the present time to reconcile the presuppositions of the problem of evil as traditionally posed (namely, that God as creator and providence is responsible for the states of affairs in the world being as they are) with what is currently considered to be the chance and necessity structure of the evolutionary and genetic processes and the accidental incidence of disease. No rationally justifiable way of understanding the character of God's creative relationship to the world exists (at any rate at present) that permits coherent questions to be asked about why God, as a responsible agent, has produced this or allowed that state of affairs in the natural order. Consequently, what is unsatisfactory is the attempt to side-line the issue of the disabled for human self-understanding into a version of the problem of evil.[15]

A second response to the challenge posed by the disabled to questions of human significance and worth is based upon the principle that difference is significant. At the end of *Science and the Modern World*, for example, Whitehead attacks both the "Gospel of Force" and the "Gospel of Uniformity." Having pointed out that "a forest is the triumph of the organization of mutually dependent species" and that "every organism requires an environment of friends," he proceeds to argue that:

> The differences between the nations and races of mankind are required to preserve the conditions under which higher development is possible.... A diversification among human communities is essential for the provision of the incentive and material for the odyssey of the human spirit.... Men require of their neighbours something sufficiently akin to be understood, and something sufficiently different to provoke attention, and something great enough to command admiration. We must not expect, however, all the virtues. We should even be satisfied if there is something odd enough to be interesting.[16]

Such a recognition of the importance of diversity does not, however, provide a basis for holding that the disabled do not raise a crucial issue for attempts to identify the significance and worth of human beings. This issue is not mitigated by pointing out that people are not like ball-bearings, or that, as is the case with licorice all-sorts, variety is the spice of life. Granted that the human community is richer because it contains violinists as well as swimmers, poets as well as engineers, rock-climbers as well as philosophers, the problem remains that it also contains a considerable number of people who may be judged to have no significant mode or modes of personal activity. It is not that while they cannot sing in tune, they are perceptive philosophers, or that while they are caring nurses, they dislike fish. The problem is that the extent of the disabilities of some people is such that it makes no sense to talk of them enjoying value-rich experiences to any significant extent, let alone of them creatively enhancing the value-experiences that they and others may enjoy. Recognition of difference in such cases is of things that may be judged to diminish instead of to enhance the human condition.

A third response suggests, implicitly if not explicitly, that so far as people are disabled, especially severely disabled, they must be excluded from consideration of the significance and worth of human beings. For a few whose responsiveness is minimal this could effectively mean that they must not be regarded as human beings. Although this is a response that many will find uncomfortable when stated openly, this is a response that lies behind some answers to the question of human value highlighted by considering the disabled. Just as one may justifiably overlook blemishes and errors in initial drafts when assessing a final product so, this response suggests, disabilities must not be taken into account in assessing the value of human being.

Such a response may be held to generalize the moral principle that John Laird, for instance, expresses when he holds that "it is never defensible to maintain that 'to be' means 'to be valuable'"[17] and, later, that:

> we distinguish between moral and sub or non-moral beings, between responsible men and women, on the one hand, and imbeciles, the lower animals and inanimate beings on the other hand.... We hold, in short, that moral beings are beings of a very high grade, privileged existents among existents not so privileged. In that sense we cannot significantly say that existence, as such, has moral properties, or that every being must be a moral being.[18]

The principle Laird enunciates is that in law, as well as in morality, the notion of responsibility is limited. Sam at twenty-one months is not responsible for his actions in the way that, in normal circumstances, he will be at twenty-one years. Again, while a person may generally be considered to have a duty to seek to save those in danger, that duty is limited to what is possible for that person to fulfil.

Does, however, the analogy apply to the case of the value of the human in relation to the disabled? What is arguable is that it does not. Leaving aside the contentious problem of where to draw the line between those people (or those conditions) which must be considered in determining the significance and worth of human beings and those which are not, the exclusion of the disabled, whether wholly or partially, from such consideration, is contrary to what has been held to be the finer instincts of humankind. Exclusion that treats the disabled like discards from a manufacturing process may be defended on the grounds that this applies to human self-understanding the preference for the fittest that characterizes the natural order. This, however, is a defence that is open to Huxley's response to advocates of so-called "evolutionary ethics," namely, that "the ethical progress of society depends, not on imitating the cosmic process, still less in running away from it, but in combatting it."[19] What may be in some respects "natural" is not necessarily good. The most satisfactory way of defining the class of authentic human beings is the genetic one. To be human is to be the child of human parents.[20] As such disabled people are to be counted as fully authentic human beings and, as Whitehead puts it, the "growth of the idea of the essential rights of human beings, arising from their sheer humanity...can be reckoned as a triumph—a checkered triumph—of the later phase of civilization."[21] The questions about the significance and worth of human beings that arise from considering the disabled are essential to comprehensive understanding of that being.

A fourth response, that may be made to the awareness of the states of the disabled, maintains that it is a mistake to take their disabilities into account in assessing a human being, for these states are temporary limitations that will be eradicated in a future post-mortem or "heavenly" mode of being. Whatever the state of their terrestrial existence, the disabled will find themselves fully "abled" in a state of subjective immortality. Such a thesis applies to the disabled Keith Ward's argument that the reality of the resurrection of Jesus justifies faith in the trustworthiness of ultimate reality:

> It is only if the resurrection is actual that the life of a crucified man can show...that Being itself is to be trusted, since death, however cruel, is not the end.... There needs to be an eschatological element to faith, an element which makes room for the vindication of the weak and suffering.[22]

Alternatively, this thesis may be seen as an application to the disabled of the evangelical tenet that through the grace of God hereafter each will be made perfect, whole and complete. It can be argued, however, that such a response to our awareness of the state of the disabled is crucially flawed.

The flaw emerges if we consider the question: But who then is the resurrected (and hence, according to the doctrine here being examined, fully abled) person? If people in a post-mortem mode of existence were to find themselves lacking disabilities that characterised the existence of some people in a previous state, to what extent would they be warranted in identifying themselves with the persons in that previous state? The model of healing may be put forward to try to justify such identification. A comment sometimes made about someone who is ill, let us call him Arthur, is that "He is not himself today." While if taken literally this is puzzling (for if Arthur is not himself, who is he?), the remark reminds us that when Arthur recovers from illness (whether physical or mental), he may well be regarded as more truly the "real Arthur" than the person who he was when he was ill. Such a judgement, however, presupposes some kind of identity and continuity with the person that Arthur was before his illness.

What is arguable is that such a model for identification and continuity is not plausible in the case of a post-mortem $Arthur_2$ who is without any of the disabilities and limitations that were always (and unalterably) the case with $Arthur_1$ in terrestrial life. Especially when the differences between the two states of personal being are major (for example, if $Arthur_2$ has modes of action, awareness, and self-awareness as well as abilities to reflect on them that were not available to $Arthur_1$), the two persons cannot reasonably be regarded as the same "Arthur" existing in different contexts, even if $Arthur_2$ inherited memories and, *mutatis mutandis*, some of the personal traits of $Arthur_1$. What we have in the case of $Arthur_2$ is the creation of a new person who has inherited some elements that were previously in $Arthur_1$ instead of a continuity of $Arthur_1$ through a process that can be compared to that of healing.

This response to the question of the significance and worth of the disabled must be rejected as profoundly demeaning to them. It suggests that their present mode of existence renders them incomplete persons and that questions of their value as persons can only be satisfactorily met when they have been provided with what they lack. If, instead, $Arthur_1$ is to be held to have significance and worth, it must be as $Arthur_1$ and not some other person who may find some memories and traits that once belonged to him. Otherwise what is being affirmed is not the value of $Arthur_1$ but of someone else.

What is also arguable is that such a post-mortem remedy for problems in this life is not satisfactory. Such a response is not satisfying to the victims nor does it supply grounds for demanding that the fairness of reality hold that those who suffer in this life will be freed of their suffering in some state hereafter. Whatever lawyers may like to pretend, some states cannot receive adequate compensation. Even less acceptable is the position that holds that however horrible is the situation now, all is fundamentally well because later things will not be horrible.

A fifth response to the issue of human worth and significance raised by taking into account the case of those who are disabled holds that disabilities must be seen as challenges to be met instead of as an intellectual problem to be solved. Maintaining that "all mysteries which mislead theory to mysticism find their rational solution in human practice," Karl Marx concludes his "Theses on Feuerbach" by asserting that "the philosophers have only interpreted the world, in various ways; the point, however, is to change it."[23] A parallel theological response is found in Wendy Farley's *Tragic Vision and Divine Compassion* where she maintains that "the radical presence of God in history" should be seen in the persistence of actions "to resist suffering, injustice, and evil."[24] According to this response disabilities should be treated like the problems presented to people on initiative courses and adventure trips. They are tests used to refine character and develop skills. Those who are challenged divide into two groups. In neither case does the response withstand scrutiny.

However, we have the disabled themselves. Some do overcome the challenges of their disabilities in impressive ways. Sarah, for example, was born without a hand. Early on those treating her advised that as much as possible she be left to find her ways of coping. She has risen to the challenges in an impressive way—from finding a way to tie an apron in a bow behind her back to becoming a world–class swimmer in her disability group. Such a response to the issue of disability only makes sense if a person's disability leaves that person with the ability to meet the challenges. It does not make sense in the case of those—and they are many—whose disabilities mean that they have no such capability. In such cases talk about meeting challenges is both ridiculous and insensitive.

The challenge may be considered to be presented not to the disabled themselves but to others who are in a position to help them. Disabilities give "able–bodied" persons opportunities both to express their compassion and to solve practical problems arising from disabilities.[25] Nevertheless, disabled people give others the chance to show their care and their skill justifies neither the condition of those who need help nor the claim that the significance and worth of disabled people lies in the way that they offer challenges to others' compassion. What is not credible, for example, is to hold that Fred's paralysis or Freda's severe mental limitations make sense and give value to Fred and Freda because of the physical and mental demands that they make upon others.

While, then, disabilities present challenges to the disabled themselves in many cases and to the temporally abled in all cases, we need to bear in mind that not all conditions can be defended as valuable for character development. An objection to the compatibility of suffering with divine providence that Laird cites can be applied to forms of disability generally:

> even if all suffering had some beneficial office, it would still be impossible to defend the amount of suffering that exists. Cancer may give an occasion for fortitude and for a certain melancholy dignity, but, in its case, anodynes are better than dignity and most of the suffering is sheer waste.[26]

Some disabilities, like some forms of suffering, destroy character—and some prevent character developing in any significant way.

Granted that the disabled, whatever the severity of their disabilities, are part of humankind, what is to be affirmed about the significance and worth of human being if each of the above five responses to disability be judged unsatisfactory? This brings us to the heart of the question of human worth. Before an attempt is made to answer it some preliminary points need to be appreciated.

The first point is that, as has already been mentioned in passing, any credible response to this question must be universally applicable. Treatment of the question is likely to be superficial if it focuses its answer too narrowly on the question as commonly presented and does not take sufficiently into account that the question tends to be presented by individuals who are convinced of the ultimate significance of being (and so of the importance of metaphysical questions), consider that they can have worth in and by themselves, and generally have both leisure to ask the question and a quality of experience that leads them to expect to find a satisfying answer to it. To be credible an answer must identify the significance and worth of every person, including those who do not ask the question, those whose experience leads them to the conviction that no satisfying answer can be found, and those who do not see any point in getting concerned about it. It must comprehend, that is, not just the Whiteheads of this world but also people like "the old bobbin' man" who said: "There are some as goes rootling and tearing about. But, Lor' bless you, sir, I gets to Saturday night as soon as any of 'em."[27]

Another preliminary point that is fundamental to this discussion, and also has already been mentioned, is the perception that the disabled as such do not constitute a distinct problem for attempts to determine the significance and worth of human beings.[28] The importance of directing attention to the disabled is that awareness of their condition helps counter the *hubris* that frequently distorts human self-understanding as people slip from thinking of themselves as the highest creatures (as known by them to exist) to regarding themselves as the highest beings that exist. Human being is finite being and is misunderstood when not recognized as such.

A third preliminary point is that any satisfactory response to the question of human significance and worth must make sense in the world that people experience themselves as inhabiting. Ian Ramsey writes about the importance of establishing the "empirical fit" of claims to understanding.[29] In these circumstances especially I find it more appropriate to see this requirement in terms of what I call "the Bright Hour Test." The "Bright Hour" are a group of ladies, most of them elderly, who regularly gather together. Although most of them have had no experience of higher education (and tend to distrust "clever talkers"), they have rich, deep, and varied knowledge of life and shrewd common sense. They may be caring and compassionate but they do not suffer from any illusions about how harsh and unrewarding life is experienced by some. When, therefore, claims that are made about the significance and worth of human beings are held to apply to those who are profoundly disabled, we need to test the credibility of those claims by the solid realism of the "Bright Hour Test": Do the claims make sense to those who know what life is like?

A final preliminary point is that consideration of the significance and worth of human beings must bear in mind the nature of personal existence. Several significant factors arise in this respect. Any satisfactory response to the question of the value of human beings must recognize, for instance, that character and context interact. People are not isolated individuals whose self-determination is independent of their surroundings. On the contrary, what they become is in part through the interaction of their intentions with their circumambient reality, both physical and social.[30] The self, furthermore, is not a permanent entity that persists unchanged through its experiences; instead from moment to moment it must be seen as the latest product of an on-going series of responses to its inheritance from the past and its envisagement of possibilities for the future. The basis of the identity of its ongoing personal character is not some unchanging core element but a combination of consistency and development of response that combines continuing acceptance of principles governing future decisions and habits formed by previous decisions with modification and novelty. Whitehead puts it that:

> 'Personal identity' is exhibited when the change in the details of fact exhibits an identity of primary character amid secondary changes of

> value.... The confusion of variety is transformed into the coordinated unity of a dominant character.... Personality is the extreme example of the sustained realization of a type of value.[31]

Nevertheless, while personal identity involves to a high degree the "memory and anticipation" essential to all life, we must recognize that the self is a reality in process.[32] As such its successive states are neither absolutely the same nor utterly different.

The self's sense of responsibility and guilt as well as social convention establish that continuity in human selfhood must exist. I recognize, for example, that *I*-now am responsible for fulfilling promises (such as a promise to repay a loan at agreed rates) that an *I*-then made some months or even years ago. If I do not fulfil such promises, *I*-now feel guilt even though *I*-now may consider that the *I*-then that made those commitments acted foolishly. In this way, the feelings of responsibility and of guilt indicate that a notion of a continuing identity is not required by social convention and convenience. The danger of social dissolution would exist if, for example, it were permissible for a person to maintain that since she or he has changed his or her mind about an action, it would be wrong to accuse him or her of being responsible for that action: the change of mind—in religious language "repentance"—in the intervening period means that the person that did the act and the person now accused of it are different persons even though, for instance, the accused has the same name and carries the same passport as the person who committed the action. The experience of being a self imposes a sense of continuity and identity: *I*-now feel that what *I*-then did is something for which *I*-now must accept liability (or, in the cases of achievements, may claim due reward).

The self does not continue through time as absolutely the same. Moments of experience perish once they have been experienced and can never be re–presented in their original state. As I recall yesterday's experiences, for instance, I may remember them as good but no longer do I experience them as mine (where to be mine is to belong to the I that *I*-now am): *I*-now experience the memory of them as being felt, not *I*-now as feeling them. Further, as I more or less vaguely recall experiences from much longer ago, I am conscious that in the intervening time the self that has become *I*-now has greatly changed—one hopes in some respects for the better. I find it embarrassing, for example, to recall the arrogant, naïve, and self-conceited student that Professor Emmet taught thirty-five years ago. As John Henry Newman said, "to live is to change, and to be perfect is to have changed often" for "whatever has life is characterized by growth, so that in no respect to grow is to cease to live."[33]

The recognition that the personal identity of a self involves memory and that a self is a state of being in process has two implications for considerations of the significance and worth of human beings. One is that a human being's awareness of his or her personal identity will be limited by the extent of her or his memory. It appears, therefore, that those who have no memory of their past cannot be considered to have a sense of personal identity. Unfortunately, some human beings have memory which is extremely limited and a few show no signs of having any conscious memory at all. This being so, any attempt to provide a universal understanding of the value of the human must take account that some human beings are not aware of their personal identity—or are not adequately aware of it. The other point is that the processive nature of the reality of being a self means that an individual's interest in the future, including subjective immortality if such exists, is, to some extent, altruistic. Just as *I*-now consider that the *I*-then that existed thirty-five years ago no longer exists as a subjective reality, even though *I*-now accept that *I*-now have inherited (for much the most part unconsciously) from that *I*-then, so *I*-now must accept that future states of *I* that inherit my current experiences will similarly distinguish themselves from *I*-now. If, for example, I were to live for another thirty-five years, the self that would exist then (and perhaps would continue into subjective immortality) would not be any more *I*-now than *I*-now consider myself to be the *I*-then of thirty-five years ago. Considerations of the significance and worth of human being need to take into account the implications of the processive nature of reality in its pre-mortem states as well as any post-mortem mode of existence, and this must include the ways in which persons change as they grow, mature, and decline. When this is done we realize that all human beings begin as radically disabled and are likely to end as such even though most in between should be classed as "temporally able-bodied."[34]

A final characteristic of the nature of human beings as personal existence that must be taken into account in considering questions of its significance and worth is its social character. Human being as personal life can only exist in relationship with others.[35] As John Macmurray puts it:

> We are not particularly personal in our baths. Hermits and castaways on desert islands have tried that way to the freedom of the personal life without very conspicuous success. The personal life is essentially a life of relations between people.[36]

Developing the point later in his Gifford Lectures, he argues that:

> we are persons not by individual right, but in virtue of our relation to one another. The personal is constituted by personal relatedness. The unit of the personal is not the 'I,' but the 'You and I.'[37]

Personal maturity develops as individuals learn to act appropriately to their context and in relation to the "others" that are around them.[38] While "the *terminus a quo* of the personal life is a helpless total dependence on the other, the *terminus ad quem* is not independence, but a mutual interdependence of equals."[39] While individuals have an intrinsic integrity that is not at the disposal of others and hence transcend others, as persons they both are known to others and become aware of their own being only as they disclose themselves to others.[40] Those, therefore, who have only limited ability to communicate with others are accordingly limited in their personal being. Consideration of the significance and worth of human beings must take account of this.

At this point, however, a clue to the answer to questions of the significance and worth of human beings begins to emerge. Recognition of the social character of human beings as personal beings makes possible the suggestion that the fundamental value of the self is in some way to be found in or through relationships with others instead of identified as something that is intrinsic to each individual. If this is the case, it becomes a communal matter. And this raises the question of the worth of those who either are or consider themselves to be outcast from community because their disabilities (whether they be intrinsic to their nature or socially imposed) prevent them entering into satisfactory and satisfying personal relationships.

In order to pursue this understanding of the value of human beings, we need to make a distinction between two terms that up to now have frequently been used in conjunction with each other as if they were roughly equivalent—as, it must be admitted, they often seem to be in common usage. These terms are "significance" and "worth." We also need to clarify their relationship, as so distinguished, to what is meant by value and by dignity.

According to the distinction which I want to use, "significance" primarily refers to the results of a person's actions and only derivatively, and so secondarily, to the person as the agent who produced those results, whether intentionally or accidentally. What a person intends to happen and what does happen as a result of an action may be different—as a person might discover on striking a match to look for a gas leak or in the case of so-called Freudian slips. Nevertheless, whatever distinctions should be made in the case of intentions and results, questions of significance concern the importance of what people perceive in what is done, and only concern the agents of those actions as a consequence. Since, therefore, judgements about the significance of actions deal with what is produced by those actions, so far as such judgements concern value, they deal with what may be said to have "contributory value," for they are concerned with the value of what those actions are perceived to contribute to the sum total of good in reality.

From this it follows that those who are responsible for deeds that bring about states of great value have, because of what they bring about, great significance, while those whose actions are limited (for example, the severely disabled) have in this respect little significance, since they bring about little of value. We must note, however, that they may have considerable significance in other respects. For example, a severely disabled person may achieve considerable significance because, while she or he never did anything remarkable themselves, his or her state led to significant advances in medical science. A dead baby in the arms of its refugee mother may have contributed minimally to the experience of value in the cosmos but a photograph of that baby published round the world may evoke humanitarian responses that are of considerable significance.

Such judgments, however, deal only (and this "only" must never be forgotten) with matters of contributory value. According to this mode of judgment, those who contribute most to society by their actions have, in respect of this kind of value, the greatest significance. This is a way of understanding value that underlies much of the radical political thought developed in the 1980s that, for good or ill, now has a powerful influence on social and political attitudes. And, it should not be overlooked, in some respects it has considerable justification. If David contributes to the common good ten times as much as Arthur, then David may be held to be correspondingly more significant than Arthur in terms of enhancing the common good.

What is a basic mistake, however, is to consider that contributory value—or what might alternatively be called earned value—is the only kind of value. As well as contributory value, what may be called "given value" or "conferred value" arises. This is the value that is given to persons, objects, states or events, not because of what those persons, objects, states, or events may contribute to others nor because of any intrinsic qualities that they may possess, but because of the way in which others regard them. While in itself an object may seem utterly trivial to people generally, someone may still confer enormous value on it—as parents sometimes discover when they have to drive back fifty miles to retrieve a tattered teddy that their child has left behind. In this way, a severely disabled individual who may be able to actualize next to nothing that has contributory value—he or she may not even show any response to what is done for them—may be the recipient of enormous given value in and through the care of others for that person.

In contrast to the contributory value that is produced by actions and is identified as their "significance," the term "worth" should thus be used to refer to the value that someone or something receives from another. As a matter of conferred value, worth may be, although it need not necessarily be, a matter of pure grace instead of a response to deserved merit. It does not belong to people or things because of some intrinsic quality that they possess or contribute to others. It results from how they are regarded by others. In other words, someone or something may in principle be held to have significance (contributory value) and worth (conferred value), or no significance but worth, or significance but no worth.

The notion of worth, as so defined, provides a way of meeting some problems that arise when value is considered wholly in terms of the notion of contributory value. It provides, for example, a basis for challenging the assumption (even if sometimes an unconscious assumption) that a person is to be judged only by what that person achieves. The consequence of adopting this assumption is seen in students who feel that they are devalued as persons when they do not get the grades that they expected, in unemployed and unemployable people who consider that they are valueless rejects because they are unproductive, in old people who apologize for being a burden on those who have to care for them, and in the case of disabled people who are conscious that they are maximal receivers and minimal providers of significant acts of contributory value. What needs to be appreciated is that, whatever the case with significance, worth is something that is given, not something that one earns by contributions. Worth is not accumulated like contributions to a pension scheme but is realized in being loved by others.

This distinction between significance and worth should be emphasized when the notion of objective immortality is considered. Standard presentations of this notion maintain, as Whitehead puts it, that God

> shares with every new creation its actual world; and the concrescent creature is objectified in God.... The image—and it is but an image—the image under which this operative growth of God's nature is best conceived, is that of a tender care that nothing be lost.... It is the judgment of a tenderness which loses nothing that can be saved. [41]

The problem with such a position is that it may well leave some individuals feeling that they have so little of significance to contribute for divine preservation that objective immortality emphasises the utter triviality of any claim to value that they might presume to assert. Forgetting the error of the *hubris* that is attached to any human claim to significance in the divine experience, they may hold that such a doctrine may appeal to the great and the good in the world's estimation but offers little or no significance for most people, let alone for an abandoned infant dying of AIDS along a refugee trail or a profoundly disabled adult who from birth has been more or less uncommunicative. Such a response, however, is only justified if, when and so far as objective immortality is considered wholly in terms of the significance (that is, of the contributory value) of persons. The situation radically changes when the issue of worth is introduced, for then it becomes possible to hold that the value of persons and the ways in which they are everlastingly held in the divine memory is not a matter of what they contribute to the divine experience but fundamentally is a matter of the divine concern for them. Each person has ultimate worth not because of what that person has achieved but because that person is cherished by God.

The importance of reference to God in relation to worth is not, however, confined to consideration of the post-mortem situation of human beings. Although no sound argument can be made for maintaining the reality of God, to deny God has uncomfortable consequences for human self-understanding. Yet, we must appreciate that the affirmation of the worth of each and every human being may be on unsure ground unless a God is present whose perfect and universal love means that each is unreservedly cherished and so given value by God.

Worth depends on the person conferring it. The objects that a child values and the character of the value that is given to them depends upon the understanding and maturity of the child. A three-year old is not likely to confer value on things as a mature Socrates might be expected to do. Further, human love, however other-directed it may wish to be, is unlikely ever to be pure and cannot avoid being limited in its extent. In consequence the worth that human love confers on those who are loved is likely to be tainted by considerations of significance (that is, of what those who are loved may contribute to the well-being of the lover) and is always inescapably partial. Divine love, however, is to be conceived as neither imperfect nor restricted. It is a pure love which unreservedly affirms the worth of the other in absolute care for that other—and, because it is God's love which affirms this worth, the worth that it confers is supreme worth. Perhaps in this way, then, instead of in terms of human rationality or human freedom or human creativity, the notions that human beings are in the image of God and that God is the parent of all should be understood. Human beings have worth not because of anything that they are in themselves (as has been noted, they seem to be a temporary and largely accidental product of an evolutionary process) nor because of anything that they may ever achieve but because God is concerned about each of them. And because God is concerned about each person, all persons have worth, even though some may justifiably feel that no one in the world cares about them.

Finally, it is in terms of this perception of the worth of human beings that their dignity must be appreciated. While some persons may properly be esteemed because of the significance of what they achieve, all persons are to be treated with dignity because of their worth. This involves recognizing their individual otherness and respecting their integrity. Whereas recognition of significance and handling with respect may be motivated by selfish aims to acquire value, conferring worth and treating with dignity is to seek to share in the love that is the creative ground of all reality.

To be realistic, however, a recognition of the relativity of value is also necessary in order to establish what level of respect is appropriate to each class of beings. This differentiation is necessary to provide a basis for establishing what is a legitimate response to such things as pests, disease, and malignant tumors. Such recognition cannot adopt a simplistic version of the claim that the highest must win over the lower without being in danger of justifying the eradication of the unneeded, the burdensome, and so on (T. H. Huxley's criticism of evolutionary ethics mentioned earlier).

What, then, is to be made of the cry for human worth? In *Persons in Relation,* John Macmurray says that "religion, as a mode of reflection, is concerned with the knowledge of the personal Other."[42] The above discussion indicates that if theism is correct in its claim that such a personal Other exists whose character as love means that each individual is cherished by God, then a basis exists for affirming that each person has not only whatever worth that is conferred upon them by fellow human beings but also unrestricted worth because they are consciously cared for by the divine. Those who adopt such a conclusion, however, must be careful that they do not thereby adopt an unwarrantably narrow view of personal nature of the divine. As Keith Ward points out:

> the greatest Christian saints, who speak of an intense love of God, also speak of the necessity of passing beyond any subject-object duality which would reduce God to the status of an object and leave God in an external relation to the loving self. They speak of the necessity of passing beyond self to achieve an experience of supreme bliss, wisdom, and compassion; and that would not be an unfamiliar concept for one who follows the Buddhist way.... Seen in this way, neither Gautama nor Jesus are sudden arbitrary eruptions of the supernatural into an otherwise closed web of natural causality. They represent the fulfilment of natural human potentialities, whereby the suprasensory is brought into living relationship with the sensory realm.[43]

What may perhaps be needed is a perception of the panentheistic character of the divine-human relationship as all-embracing love;[44] what must be included is the perception that this love affirms the worth of each and every human being. The human cry for worth is satisfied by the divine in a totally inclusivistic way. No human being is excluded from the divine love and therefore no human being lacks the ultimate worth that divine love confers.

NOTES

1. John Macquarrie, "Theological Reflections on Disability," in *Religion and Disability: Essays in Scripture, Theology, and Ethics*, edited by Marilyn E. Bishop (Kansas City: Sheed and Ward, 1995), pp. 30-32.

2. *Ibid.*, p. 32. See also Alfred North Whitehead, *Process and Reality: An Essay in Cosmology*, corrected edition. ed. D. R. Griffin and D. W. Sherburne (New York: The Free Press, 1978), p. 340, 344; John B. Cobb, Jr., *God and the World* (Philadelphia: The Westminster Press, 1969), pp. 46-65).

3. Whitehead, *Process and Reality*, p. 350f.

4. *Ibid.*, p. 350; cf. p. 346.

5. H. Richard Niebuhr, *The Meaning of Revelation* (New York: Macmillan, 1941), p. 77, 150.

6. Schubert M. Ogden, *The Reality of God and Other Essays* (London: SCM Press, 1967), p. 140f.

7. Georg Wilhelm Friedrich Hegel, *Lectures on the History of Philosophy, The Lectures of 1825–1826*. Vol. 3: Medieval and Modern Philosophy, ed. R. F. Brown, translated by R. F. Brown and J. M. Stewart with the assistance of H. S. Harper (Berkeley, Los Angeles, Oxford: University of California Press, 1990), p. 245.

8. Jean-Paul Sartre, *Existentialism and Humanism*, edited by Philip Mairet (London: Methuen, 1948), p. 26.

9. Peter C. Hodgson, *Winds of the Spirit: A Constructive Christian Theology* (Louisville, Ken.: Westminster John Knox Press, 1994), p. 180.

10. Alfred North Whitehead, *Essays in Science and Philosophy* (New York: Greenwood Press, 1968), p. 121.

11. David A. Pailin, *A Gentle Touch: From a Theology of Handicap to a Theology of Human Being* (London: SPCK, 1992).

12. *Ibid.*, pp. 4-6.

13. Hodgson, *Winds of the Spirit*, p. 199.

14. Reinhold Niebuhr, *The Nature and Destiny of Man: A Christian Interpretation*, Vol. 1, "Human Nature" (London: Nisbet, 1941), pp. 286f, 292; cf. 182f.

15. See David A. Pailin, *Probing the Foundations: A Study in Theistic Reconstruction* (Kampen, The Netherlands: Kok Pharos, 1994), ch. 9.

16. Alfred North Whitehead, *Science and the Modern World* (Cambridge, England: Cambridge University Press, 1926), p. 258.

17. John Laird, *Mind and Deity* (London: George Allen and Unwin, 1941), p. 203.

18. *Ibid.*, p. 216f.

19. Thomas H. Huxley, *Evolution and Ethics and Other Essays* (London: Macmillan, 1895), p. 83; cf. p. 31.

20. Pailin, *A Gentle Touch*, pp. 54–56.

21. Alfred North Whitehead, *Adventures of Ideas* (Cambridge, England: Cambridge University Press, 1933), p. 15.

22. Keith Ward, *Religion and Revelation: A Theology of Revelation in the World's Religions* (Oxford: Clarendon Press, 1994), p. 252.

23. Karl Marx and Friedrich Engels, *On Religion*, with an introduction by Reinhold Niebuhr (New York: Shocken Books, 1964), p. 71f.

24. Wendy Farley, *Tragic Vision and Divine Compassion: A Contemporary Theodicy* (Louisville, Ken.: Westminster/John Knox Press, 1990), p. 132.

25. *Cf.* Nancy Eiesland and Rebecca Chopp, *The Disabled God: Toward A Liberatory Theology of Disability* (Nashville, Tenn.: Abingdon Press, 1994) pp. 8 and 24.

26. Laird, *Mind and Deity*, p. 178.

27. Whitehead, *Essays in Science and Philosophy*, p. 20.

28. *Cf.* Pailin, *A Gentle Touch*, pp. 58-63.

29. *Cf.* Ian Ramsey, *Models and Mystery* (Oxford: Oxford University Press, 1964), pp. 17, 38–40.

30. *Cf.* Robert Cummings Neville, *The Highroad Around Modernism* (Albany, NY: State University of New York Press, 1992), p. 189f.

31. Whitehead, *Essays in Science and Philosophy*, p. 85f.

32. *Ibid.*, p. 91.

33. John Henry Newman, *An Essay on the Development of Christian Doctrine* (London: Longmans, Green, and Co., 1890), pp. 40, 185.

34. Cf. John Macmurray, *Persons in Relation* (London: Faber and Faber, 1961), p. 62.

35. See Neville, *The Highroad Around Modernism*, p. 104f.

36. John Macmurray, *Reason and Emotion* (London: Faber and Faber, 1962), p. 96.

37. Macmurray, *Persons in Relation*, p. 61; cf. p. 69f.

38. *Ibid.*, p. 64f.

39. *Ibid.*, p. 66.

40. Cf. Hodgson, *Winds of the Spirit* (SCM Press, London: 1994) p. 129; John Macmurray, *Interpreting the Universe* (Faber and Faber, London: 1933), p. 134f.

41. Whitehead, *Process and Reality*, p. 345f.

42. Macmurray, *Persons in Relation*, p. 168.

43. Ward, *Religion and Revelation*, p. 334f.

44. *Cf.* Pailin, *Probing the Foundations*, pp. 116–132.

Four

TOWARD A PHILOSOPHY OF LOSS

Charles C. Conti

In philosophizing loss, I want to suggest a line of thought (1) which is compatible with the prevalent personalist postulate of "connaturality," emphasizing our social complicity, but (2) is more radical than the idea that persons are merely "natural with" others, and so act as moral communicants. I want to suggest that the compositional structure of consciousness, how consciousness came into being, including how "the self" is formed, involves something more drastic than that personal identity is a socially transacted phenomenon, or that the person-concept is allotropic and capable of existing in two forms simultaneously, the public and the private. I want to claim that consciousness involves a negation of ego-identity, must learn to live with loss at the center of its being. A couple of aphorisms help make the point. One is an ancient Jewish proverb: "A person is not whole who is not conscious of a lack." The other is from Dietrich Bonhoeffer, German theologian, who in his *Letters and Papers from Prison* wrote: only in death do "we think...about the people...we should not like to live without...It is only then that we realize how closely our own lives are bound up with other people's...how little we are separate entities."[1]

In the course of explaining how the innovative work of Jacques Lacan supports the remark that "the centre of lives is actually outside ourselves," I want to indicate how the extremely subtle issue of personal identity might be used to rethink a philosophy of language. If, as Feuerbach said (quoting Luther) a world of faith is of unlimited subjectivity, and if at the heart of subjectivity is not mirror images but symbols of ineffability, mystery, and even loss, then the sort of "negative theology" we find in Lacan may be capable of releasing a constructive theory of language precisely by deconstructing standard denotational models.

Let us begin with Lacan's account of the mirror-stage: sometime in the interval of intimacy which occurs in the development of the child between six and eighteen months, the child experiences its body as fragmented, likely the result of weaning, and becomes able to recognize its image as if in a mirror. Not a literal mirror; the self-imaging, and the child's fascination with it, is less a reflection of itself than an image it gets of itself from another. But well before six months, experiments show the new-born is able to imitate its parent's smiling face, a game of mimicry as between two syncopated partners. The influence is two-way. The Mother picks up any form of recognition of her influence, extending sentience to the neonate. To the adoring Mother, the child's labiality becomes profoundly answerable.

For Lacan, such social miming marks the beginning of self-awareness. The mirroring face smiles at the child, and the Mother hopes her response will be seen by the child as an invitation to respond in kind. So the child picks up the cue, the one it innocently gave, and, more often than not, what (according to Dr. Spock) begins as mere indigestion, when the child's face breaks into a broad smile, takes on added social significance. Such games of recognition are, for Lacan, far from trivial. Mirror images offer the child an identification with another which is a reflectional reception of itself. The child readily re-cognizes itself in the other. No longer an "in-itself," the self becomes a "split"-self. It "sees" self in the mirror-Mother. Such "reflections" mark the transformation of the subject from what Freud described as a literal extension of the Mother's body, to an image of itself outside itself: still a part of the Mother, but no longer physically attached. The child is now objectified in the face of the other, and it can affect the Mother's face, as the Mother affected it.

A problem exists in the mirror image. The child may find it easier to recognize the Mother's face than its own. This is because we are less an object to our self than to others; more accustomed to seeing the face of others than observing our own face. This is a disquieting fact of personal identity and we carry it with us the rest of our life. Deflected images create a permanent sense of open insecurity. Deflected identity is receptional identity. We become reflectional beings, beyond mere self-reflection. You are more transparently object to me; and the same subjectifying process holds true in return.

Another fated ambiguity exists in the mirror metaphor. A mirror-image can either represent the person as the person appears to oneself (like those fleeting glimpses we catch of our self in the dirty pane of the underground train) or how we appear to others (as when adults put on a "social face" to enhance their receptivity by others). But we enhance our receptivity to others by recognizing the medianship of others, acknowledging their mirror unto us. This is because the subject is never fully "object" to itself, since it is only "by" those others being a subject to our self that we ourselves become a subject in the first place. Lacan's remark about being "subjected to" the gaze of another is relevant: "the subject is subject only from being subjected to the field of the Other."[2] In short, the subject subjects. Personal identity is of the lend/lease variety.

For Lacan, this "subjecting" is not just a heuristic device; the image of the self is permanently split, irreparably so. This is not only because of a biological deficiency (neonates cannot sustain life outside the womb without a support system); psychologically, it is because the mirror image is reflexive in a literal sense. It offers a precise copy. Genuine spontaneity is lost. "It" becomes self-reflective. So philosophy was born (Lacan warns) in the introverted image; in the introversion of meaning or inspection of the signs of intro-spection. This is because the image in the mirror is devoid of social content or human responsiveness. A mirror image mocks the "self" as its own narcissistic twin. Descartes called it reflection and saw it was good; *contra* God who saw it was not good for man to be alone, so made Adam a helpmate.

In Cartesian introspection, the image of "the self" becomes the object of its own possession, and self-conscious. Descartes assumed the human being was an autonomous subject, separable from others and even the conditions of its own cognizance. When consciousness looked inside itself, it found a subject fully present to itself, self-identical with itself. Subjectivity became object to itself. For Descartes, the human subject "owns" itself. To philosophers of action such "ownership" is achieved by forfeiture, due to lack of external exposure. Lacan's "mirror-stage" undermines this Cartesian subject. The child sees itself in the mirror and identifies itself with the "object" there, while also identifying itself here as a "subject"-self. This fundamental alienation or duality lies at the base of human identity. Are we "there" in the mirror image, or "here," inside our self? Since the answer is "both," it undermines the interior view of the self as uncovering the rock bottom of consciousness in itself.

In the beginning then was the mirror-stage, a strong desire for the image of a body to be repossessed by the (M)other. Missing that elemental unity, the child is at an acute loss and wishes to reclaim its lost intimacy, emplacement. In Freud, this reidentification was linked with the desire for death or pure embeddedness. An entombing womb represents the homeostasis of reunification, "peace, perfect peace," which, in another ominous image, descended from the Father above. But this descending scythe was ever ready to castrate the child's expanding consciousness, as in Edgar Alan Poe's "The Pit and the Pendulum." What takes the place of the entombing womb or the castrating Father in Lacan is subtler. It is the transformation of the erotic relation into a fantasy-desire which warns us off narcissistic introspection. A transformation both radical and complex takes place when the subject assumes an image. Consciousness becomes embarrassed; self-conscious in the presence of the other. Consciousness is henceforth split in twain. By "socializing" Freud's pleasure principle (*Lustprinzip*) Lacan expelled consciousness from the Freudian womb and propelled it into the symbolic. Another way to say this is that he, Lacan, staved off the attempt to reclaim the missing mother by playing the knave, a language-rogue.

Notice, a substitution has occurred. The subject is separated from the love of the Mother, as well as alienated from his or her human property, the capacity to be reflected in the image of a responding face. It perceives itself. The image takes on a false reference-point "outside" the self. Since the image itself can't be touched, only the mirror, the image of self indexes an "imaginary register." (Put again, the child loses control of the appeasement of its desires which hitherto the Mother has provided, so fantasizes the loss.) But even in the nurturing stage, the mother does not so much mirror the child directly to itself (as in Winnicott's account) as grant an image-expectation which her absence immediately deflects.

Lacan reminded us of Freud's *fort/da* game, where the child's spool is thrown from the cot, then reeled in: "there" one minute; "gone" the next. Charles Winquist described this act of withdrawal in quasi-theological terms. "The mirror image can be thought of as a referential fantasy or *imago* for a transcendental unity of apperception that is outside of the subject."[3] Philosophers look for "the real" behind the referential fantasy; while theologians purport to find it in a "love that wilt not let me go." Hypostasized in an image centrally located "outside" the self; alternatively, incarcerated in an abiding image whose constancy mocks genuine intersubjectivity, the subject becomes alienated from truly interactive sociality.

Here we see the psychological equivalent of that aseity which trapped God in its own perfection. In Aquinas's system, God became "fullness of being" or "being itself," *ipsum esse*. Ipseity or aseity stems from the Latin *a se* emphasizing "being for oneself"; the equivalent of that solipsism which is also self-reflective, *solus ipse*. Significantly, the Levinasian tradition substitutes illeity for aseity. *Illeity*, from the French *il y a* or "thereness," emphasizes third-party reference (usually by ostensive indication). This reveals the longing for relation from being addressed by another. Levinas describes it as "the trace of the other." Buber found it representative of the summoning mode; this by way of contrast with the obsession of self-reference or even self-reliance, by which William James critiqued "God's famous inventory of perfections."

> God... as any orthodox text-book will tell us, is a being existing not only *per se*, by himself, as created beings exist, but *a se*, or from himself; and out of this "aseity" flow most of his perfections. He is, for example, necessary; absolute; infinite in all respects; and single. He is simple, not compounded of essence and existence, substance and accident, actuality and potentiality, or subject and attributes, as are other things. He belongs to no genus; He is inwardly and outwardly unalterable; He knows and wills all things, and first of all His own infinite self, in one indivisible eternal act. And He is absolutely self-sufficing, and infinitely happy. Now in which one of us practical Americans here assembled does this conglomeration of attributes awaken any sense of reality: And if in no one, then why not? Surely because such attributes awaken no responsive active feelings and call for no particular conduct of our own. How does God's "aseity" come home to you?[4]

To bring it "home," render God more conceivable, a yet more radical reading of *illeity* is offered by Gillian Rose. The expiation of the new onto-theology is uniquely suited to the silence of God because it echoes to the *il* or *ille* of "he" or "she." This is a proper form of "dialogic" address in the absent presence of God, since "he" or "she" represents the anonymity of engendered relations and at the same time allows for personal "forms of address." In the dirempted middle "broken unto you" (portrayed in Rose's book *The Broken Middle*) *ipseity* contrasts with the "there-ness" of *illeity*, a middle (of silent) distance broken by the echo of personal pronouns, "I," "you," and "I/thou." This is reminiscent of Buber. Against those who deem him to have externalized the "Eternal Thou" to justify his anthropological presupposition, Buber turned it around. "But in the end, man, having attained to clear knowledge, must recognize that every alleged colloquy with the divine was only a soliloquy, or rather a conversation with various strata of the self."[5] This warns "the self" from that vicious form of imprisoning experienced by the classical God of self-sufficiency, caught in its own originary. The language of colloquy marks an appeal to be heard, and is seductive. In the debate between Barth and Brunner, the *analogia relationis* or "analogy of relationships" came to play a vital role in neo-Reformation theology. As male to female so creature to creator.

lleity, for Rose, redresses the need to communicate while simultaneously reinforcing the ethical. This further canvasses the relation between morality and theology. We grasp an essential element of the pathway of the human spirit in its emergent form if and when we regard it from the standpoint of the changes introduced in relationships which occur when we pass from the merely ethical to the moral. "It [*sc. illeity*] makes the word God be pronounced, without letting 'divinity' be said...." "Thou," being addressed, is to a reverentially sacred "other." Farrer would agree with the sentiments that morality is that "through which the Infinite leaves a trace in cognition." For the "I" of Thou is a spoken Word. And after the word became flesh, after *logos*, finite words.

This confirms the importance of using the proper model for conceiving God. The logical result of Descartes's internal cogitator is a Being who basks in the mirror of its own perfection and is the apex of being. Such a hypostasis of being (as discussed in my *Metaphysical Personalism*) does little justice to the active criteria by which we judge things to be "real" or accede to personal identity.

Philosophically speaking, self-referential theories of language experience similar limitations. They grant insufficient motility. Realism looks for the lost object-referent, an exact replica of things as they are—one hears talk of the substance behind the shadow or, with Kant, of things in themselves—while idealism is captivated by the entire process of *percipere*, mesmerized by its own powers of perception. On Lacan's reading (deliberately designed to shock), realists were weaned too early, so spend the rest of their life looking for the missing object, while idealists remain convinced that the flow of reality is somehow dependent on their ability to receive it.

That this metaphor, of a "mirror image," is not only about psychology, but doubles as a commentary on how language "courts" things, is brought out nicely by R. D. Laing in *The Divided Self*. "There are some people...who never fully real-ize themselves." A man might say he is "unreal"; "made of glass, of such transparency and fragility that a look directed at him splinters him to bits and penetrates straight through him."[6] And when we seek internal repairs, or look within to discover our real or true self, "there can be only our footprints." We are mindfully wary of Hume. The fragility of "the look" also plays a part in Sartre's work. To look is not to see, but to recognize the capability to be looked at.

Unlike Laing, Lacan's human subject is not a "divided self" that ideally in a different society could be made whole, but a self "only actually and necessarily created within a split—a being that can only conceptualize itself when it is mirrored back to itself." Stronger still; no human being can become a subject outside this split. The mirror image is more than a pedagogic device to shatter verbal realism or to cure social divisiveness; the form of the shared-self in the mirror image generates a splitness which has pseudo-empirical credibility. What looks like a real object but whose mimicry informs us it is only a mirror image, can, on analysis, be seen to represent the controls of the apperceiving mind, controls which, for better or worse, are committed to the reappropriation of reality by placing the images under the seer's control. In this way, the mirror image marks the entry into the realm of the imaginary. According to Jacqueline Rose, the image ostensibly locates us in an order "outside" us to which we are constantly beholden to refer. Here we have a literal image of our incapacity to seize "the real self," as well as an image which helps us imagine its own limitation, and so gives birth to, first the symbolic, then the imaginary realms. This fosters the shift from image to the imaging ability itself, since the shifting form of the image in the mirror serves not to reinforce a reality-factor. The mirror does not tell us how it is, only how things appear. Talk of "things in themselves" is, on this score, a vain attempt to get behind the mirror into the wonderland of embellished images. Ego-isolate, the self offers a false front. The self is now sick and divided.

Philosophically, the consciousness which beholds itself and asks the mirror to attest to the truth is offered a referential lie because it is a self-referential truth. Asked what it thinks of itself, the mirror-image cannot help but be complicitious. The mirror serves to enhance the conscious mode which hails itself, narcissistically. Better to halt the "object" of observation in its tracks by turning a blind eye or by "forgetfulness." The truth of the naming subject, who is not yet a language-speaker but only a language-seeker, is not to be found in logicizing an-other referent; something to name or someone to call upon, a present help in time of persistent need. We need presence without insistence; persona without compulsion. For Lacan, no help exists; no concrete referent for the symbol. In the absence of the concrete signified, the missing object comes to haunt the subject as its missing rib.

Opening the "inscape" of language to deeper imagery, Julia Kristeva advocates "the bright and fragile amatory idealization." Her work, entitled "The Black Sun," offers light without representation, insistence without presence; the shadow cast on the fragile self by the loss of the other. Lacan too advocates the "rivenness" of speech. He accepts the Saussurian distinction between signifier and signified, but credits the signifiers as carrying more significance than the signified. "The signified is constantly sliding under the signifier." Lacan is saying that what does the referring, the word, is more important than that to which language refers or is beholden, "things." He cites Humpty Dumpty in support and claims to want "to reinstate... the sovereign liberty displayed by Humpty Dumpty when he reminds Alice that he is master of the signifier, even if he isn't the master of the signified in which his being took on its form."[7] This represents a move from nomenclaturism—acting "in the name of the Father" where Adam is invested with the authority to call the animals and name them—to the abstract or the symbolic; from "names as tags" to linguisticism or "beyond" labels. The signified is caught in a web of signification. A "web" has many-fixing points as a mirror has infinite reflexivity.

Given the mirror image does not profitably divide into a worthy counterpart but only a clone of our own face, the mirror reminds us that something is missing, a real other. To try to replace the missing "object" with literalism or verbal realism is to err philosophically. Because of the developing subjectivity to which it relates, given that subjectivity is permanently split, the signified is only ever half-formed in refracted or diffracted allusions. Poetically, no word is without its penumbra or fringe. Limitless signifiers remake the world. We remark on things using language markers. Written with a hyphen, the word "re-mark" appears five times in Edith Wyschogrod's slender two-and-a-half-page "Introduction" to Lacan, entitled "Re-marks."

What kind of re-mark releases the signification of the signifier? Is it a verbal mirror offering a picture theory of reality, *à la* the early Wittgenstein, or hues of meaning, shaded and nuanced, as in community use? It is closer to the latter. For Lacan, language functions more like the unconscious with its free associations, verbal slips, hidden or double meanings, and even mistakes the propositional riders for imagistic retakes. He coined a word, *méconaissance*, to convey the importance of mis-cognitions, limiting the purchase of cognitive theories of reference. We do not see through a glass darkly and only eventually face to face. Nor do we rely on those "blessed givens" much beloved of English philosophers, picking up sensory cues from the far side of noumenal reality. We do not re-cognize what we already know, appealing to innate or *a priori* truths. We do not see through the unconscious blindfolded, as Freud assumed, or through a veil of deep, dark, aberrant desires. We "see" by drawing back the curtain of desire, draping it with seven seductive veils, more provocative than any form of frontal nullity, that denudification of language which assumes the trichotomous "true, false, or meaningless" covers the entire range of reference.

This does not replace, but supplements, the orthodox interpretation of Freud. In discussing the unconscious, Freud is reputed to have said, "Where the 'Id' is, there shall the 'Ego' be." Lacan is saying: Where an "it" is signified, the ego of the signifier superabounds and is even more to be found. In Freud, ego must learn to triumph over and replace the Id. "Where the Id is, there I will be."

For Freud, the Ego must "found" itself on the darker shores of Eros; if not that, it will likely flounder on the shoals of repressed sexuality. Lacan wants the Ego to come to recognize its origins in a self-dissolving process. For him, we gain our soul or the spirit of personhood by giving up the object of Id-ification. This loss of "object-ness"—quiddity or "thinghood" in an older school of philosophy—has deep significance for the entire signifying process. It resists the patrician idea that below the floor of ordinary confused grammar lies an ideal logical form and equally the idea that any worthy philosophy of language must be typically "thingy." What is therefore "unassimilable" in Freudian theory—how projection can positively contribute to the developing ego where no act of sexual repression is present—is better accounted for in Lacan (1) in the recognition that the passage of the mind from the mirror stage to the imaginary is a linguistic phenomenon or linguistic rite of passage; (2) in the realization that the complementarity of others, how we engage them, need not be sexual but social, conceptual, even quasi-ontological. What engenders language is, for Lacan, not a gendered other, but simply an "other." This is part of the meaning of that saying, "there is no other of the other." No absolute other to effect salvific repairs on the fragmented soul so that we can ever say "underneath are the everlasting arms."

Whereas normal speech tries to tie each signifier down to a single signified, Lacan, by contrast, championed a language of free association which exults in double and multiple meanings, utilizing puns, word-play, and paradoxes to defy the repressive, circumspect practices of our normal speech. This takes with it the *unum nomen unum nominatum* fallacy—one name per thing named. A poetics of witticism (*jeu d'esprit*) and jokery (*calembour*) gives utterance to the hidden desires of the unconscious. Lacan spoke of "the malicious grace of the mind free from care" and, as an example of that glee, coined a word, *poubellication*, suggesting that the serious practice of publication is like placing rubbish in a dustbin, *poubelle* in French. And when he feared his school in Paris was becoming too "institutionalized," he promptly disbanded it.

"Linguistic play" is not only a redeeming feature of language, a salve for that overbearing sincerity one finds in religion and sanitized philosophy, but is an indispensable part of the entire conceptual process. Lacan's philosophy of language offers a fruitful response to Freud's discovery that unconscious desires have their own form of language not readily translatable into conventional rhetoric or linear thinking. Freud spoke of repression, transference, dream emissions, and other escape—vulva—turning inside out the pocket-cloaca of hidden meanings and finding only spent up images (giving feminists due cause to protest the dehiscent imagery). Lacan argued that "the language of unconscious desire, which expresses itself in dreams and symptoms, works dialectically in terms of riddles." Language is diachronic and changeable, neither perverse nor chronically in need of referential repairs, as it was for Bertrand Russell and the Logical Positivists earlier in the twentieth century.

Lacan returned language to the people, and remythologized speech. "It was certainly the Word that was in the beginning, and we live in its creation, but it is the action of our spirit that continues this creation by constantly renewing it." How close is this to the poet's talk of finding "a broader spiritual resonance" in language?[8] And how far from Ted Hughes's *Crow*? "In the beginning was the word"; it said "Caw"—caw for carnage. Crow looked for the grammarian scraps to feed off. It was not that way in the beginning. In the beginning was the mirror-stage. It brought creation not "out of nothing," but by the reciprocal word, itself dialogical: "Let there be...; and there was".... co-namers and enframers, occupants who make worlds by making versions. These versions turn on the visionary yield of our concepts. Neither a war on words nor silence worship of the "beyond" of mysticism. The world of words create the world of things. Words enframe or encode a "human" world. The world "worlds." This is a view of "world" as rich and varied as the language by which we describe it. "World" as construct.

Lacan dispelled, in a single move, the prejudicial assumptions of both traditional psychology, with its repressive forces of hidden selfhood, and conventional philosophy, with its representational hopes of picture images. He effectively denied that "Id" constitutes a den of unruly animal drives without rhyme or reason. The unconscious desires (according to Lacan) unfold according to a language which is even more sophisticated than the discourse of the conscious intelligence. For, to repeat, the mirror does not give "thing"-presentations, only a point of reference, from ourselves. More, Lacan taught that the subject only becomes a subject, an autonomous other, in the distension of its need. Desire not only resists satiation, it embraces the looseness of symbol, flirtatiously. Whereof we cannot speak, we are well advised to let unconsciousness in. A hidden desire lurks in such sentential rites. To "name" is not to access the *Ding an sich,* but to allude to those "asemantic escholalias" so typical of the unconscious, a word which expresses itself in sound utterances, so arranges the wild flowers of glossolalia found in abundance in ordinary speech.

Lacan's weaning of the conceptual neonate into signifying images comes by way of a form of self-denial. Just as the child does not reclaim the parent's missing presence by re-appropriation of the symbol of nurture, neither does the child pine for the *soma* of the missing mother. Julia Kristeva coined a word to connote the symbolic rejection of the object, "abjection." The word conveys fascination and impossibility. It is precisely the ambiguity of the "abject" that distinguishes it from ordinary objects. The abject is that which "disturbs identity, system, order"; it is the "in-between, the ambiguous, the composite."[9] When the subject "ob-jects" to the lost object without quite knowing what is lost, what (exactly) that object is, it assumes the state of abject misery, is "cast out," which experience of disturbing self-exclusion is expressed as "abjection" or personal loss. Kristeva writes: "I expel myself, I spit myself out, I abject myself with the same motion through which 'I' claim to establish myself."[10]

Not by straightforward representation, then, is the gap between signifier and signified closed down or transposed into the art of versicals. Kristeva's reading of the movement from the unconscious is less by way of language than by redolent images. It is a gaining which is achieved by a letting go, a vile letting go, a forceful self-ejection so to speak, "abjection," a vomiting expulsion, an abhorrence of facticity. We must learn to "abject" ourselves as our own love-object, and become "suspicious of all master narratives."[11]

As such, all heresies begin with the fetishism of the signifier. That includes the icons of idolatry and the identity of first principles. Having forgotten their own dialogical roots, "humans...reinterpreted traditional religious symbols in their own image. God was no longer the covenant partner, dialogue with whom assembled earth and sky and mortals, but became a subject manipulating the world, who could in turn be manipulated—a fetish." In effect, persons reduced themselves to "subjects of an apotheosized Subject [a God], exercising his power on them for a unilaterally chosen goal."[12] However, this is not so. The suffering, broken, consoling language which arises from the archeology of the soul provides the truer alchemy of meaning. It is not the truth as verified or falsified or idealized, but displacement of the "truth" about writing. In the symbolic, we are trying to release, yet sustain, the expression of an intangible loss. For Freud, we are reinscribing horrors we are trying to repress with a mythology which borders on the pathological. For Lacan, what opens beneath textuality is not the phobic jaws of the castrating Father or the search for a missing authority, but a parodic "under language" which displaces the truth of writing, polysemy, "the unavoidable diaspora of written signs." Meaning, like the wandering Jew, seeks a homeland. Unlike the powerful Moses of monotheism, it is indeterminate. "The function of language is not to inform, but to evoke."[13]

Truth, like the Mother's presence, becomes "standoffish" in Lacanian symbolics. Recast in our original metaphor, no exact mimetic reference can exist in the mirror image, and no nurture. As such, any theory of language based on exact replicas is bound to fail. Like the Mother's communiques, the meaning lies in the labiality, even liability, of words. This is a kind of babble which, according to George Steiner, awaits response. The symbolic marks the possibility of representational multifacity or "iconicity," not object-fixation or denotative purity or even depictive relief (as Janet Martin Soskice bedizens the function of metaphor in her work).

Steiner, master wordsmith, highlights the fundamental irreducibility of the text. Earlier, the philosopher Friedrich Waismann, used the "open texture" of the language of description to force Logical Positivism to acknowledge the valoric way we describe things. No "paraphrastic study" in worn-out pentameter to lament "the intolerable wrestle with words and meanings" on behalf of which T.S. Eliot conducted a "raid on the inarticulate." No poverty at all, as Eliot's rich storehouse of words in "Four Quartets" attests. In poetry, we are left with "the untranslatability of an iconic presence" which, in Steiner's estimation, is irreducible into alternative vocabularies, a brighter, clearer residue lying at the bottom of the poetical pool.

The healing powers of the natural word take over from the "Father-imagery" of philosophical strife and oppositionality. Disavowing totalitarian images—the phallocratism of "monocentric totemism"—Lacan spoke of acting "the-name-of-the-Father," transmogrified over the years into a pseudo-name by being written as a single noun. For the binary oppositions of word and world, Lacan substituted a creative *Logos* whose cup runneth over, and so converts "the book of nature" into a literary tome-poem.

It should by now be evident that when Lacan says "the unconscious is structured like a language," he is not arguing that "the unconscious" teaches us abhorrence for "word-exactions," as Eliot foolishly tried to "unsay" in "Burnt Norton," a thesis which imploded under the weight of words. Lacan is claiming that the origins of language lie in the eternal longing, even co-belonging, of the unconscious; and that the unconscious speaks an insatiable desire to love and be loved. As the symbolic is to the imaginary, so language transcends the world by proxy, not by direct, dim, or distant approximation. Lacan shows us how to "go beyond language" without violating the limits of language by going "behind" language. His "retreat" does not have the same mutinous element as Steiner who advocated "logically bastard modes" in assaying a "retreat from the Word." Using the sonorities of music and the resonances of poetry to decorate, bewilder, and enhance all at once, Steiner sought a *tertium quid* between the mute radiance of realism and the mawkish sounds of "word exactions." In Lacan, what is felt as a sense of loss—trivially, the inability to put things into words—is more accurately an incomplete sense of "the self." So it is not that "thick" language must be restructured in order to have the "referential motility" thinner theories of language naturally possess (like Lucky's unrepressed "word-salad" speech in Beckett's *Waiting for Godot* attests or e.e. cumming's word play). We need not compare surface slickness to hidden streams of stealth in contrasting poetical and philosophical styles. Nor is Lacan saying that language should be structured more like the unconscious in being less confident about the purchase of its concepts and encouraged to use poetry to better cope with the imprecisions of life. He is claiming that the truth of language is dysfunctional and that such disintegration alone has the power to save us from the power-barons of propositional correctness. Such language saves us by releasing us unto eternal desire, thereunto the "other." The "eternal question" posed in the dialogue of lovers is, "What value has my desire for you?"[14] If this is right and language is the search for a displaced love-object, it follows that the way of language is the way of amorous love, *via amarosa*, since in the search for love, the monadic self gives way to a nomadic ego, an ego which comes to rest or finds a home in colloquy. Martin Buber underscored Wittgenstein's insight:

> Speech in its ontological sense was all times present wherever men regarded one another in the mutuality of I and Thou; wherever one showed the other something in the world in such a way that from then on he or she began really to perceive it; wherever one gave another a sign in such a way that he or she could recognize the designated situation as [s]he had not been able to before; wherever one communicated to the other his or her own experience in such a way that it penetrated the other's circle or experience and supplemented it from within, so that from now on his or her perceptions were set within a world as they had not been before. All this flowing ever again into a great stream of reciprocal sharing of knowledge—thus came to be and thus is the living We, the genuine we, which, where it fulfils itself, embraces the dead who once took part in colloquy and now take part in it through what they have handed down to posterity.[15]

The "wording"-process does not lead us to the structuration or even to the deconstructive capability of words, but that "the way of love and desire" marks a profound shift from ego-centism to ex-centrism, moving us from a pre-possessed to a decentered self. This is because love both secures and unstabilizes through its identification with another. Gillian Rose, using themes of dis-possession, warned against self-emplotment:

> A soul which is not bound is as mad as one with cemented boundaries. To grow in love-ability is to accept the boundaries of oneself and others, while remaining vulnerable, woundable, around the bounds. Acknowledgement of conditionality is the only unconditionality of human love.[16]

For Rose, the only unconditional truth of human relationships is the fact of the soul's pilgrimage of conditionedness. Not only "soul-talk," the language of "unconditional love" is also the language of religion and co-morality. An ego in love has captured the sense of being enthralled by another. For Levinas, building on this binding, the call to infinite love, to *caritas*, does not devastate the self. *Caritas* awakens the self. The transcendental "in" of the concept "Infinite" qualifies the "finite." It does not "name" God. It designates the depth to which the affections must go, or empty themselves, to incarnate "the self" without conscious sacrifice. The concept of "the Infinite" infinitizes affectional love.[17] It does this by evoking adoration, uplifts by invocation.

Religious imagery creates a logical space sufficient to accommodate self and others in a trinity of perfection: "body, soul, and paraclete as one." Paraclete, the soul of our co-belonging. It announces "the comforter has come." Where else, or where more provocatively does this transformation take place but by dispossessing our material beliefs? For flesh does not seek incorruption; it covets only a "return to the body where I was born," a hallowed place, a parenthetical space. According to Allen Ginsberg, creating an interval or space between the ego and the self is redemptive, where reflexivity is directed at something other than itself, whereupon (affecting a slight substitution) "the soul comes joyful to the 'I'."[18] Here the singular form of address, the "I," reclines in second-person repose. Graced by another, consciousness becomes "We." This is the blessed "We" of Buberian colloquy. For Buber, like Foucault, sex is a profoundly semantical act because it is subjected to communication. It drives us into acts of solicitation; into the arms of another. But the act of communication is an art; it does not guarantee its object, nor any object for that matter. By self-dispossession, we hail the advent of the other, and allow for the desire of being desired. This alters the reference-range of language:

> Language never existed before address; it could become monologue only after dialogue broke off or broke down. The early speaker was not surrounded by objects on which he imposed names, nor did adventures befall him that he caught with names: the world and destiny became language for him only in partnership. Even when in a solitude beyond the range of call the hearerless word pressed against the throat, this word was connected with the primal possibility, that of being heard.[19]

It is the celebratory sense of *jouissance*, a joy bubbling up from within the need for identification with another—of which sexuality is its most obvious symbol—which woos the lost object. Sex becomes a symbol of wholeness: sigh and sign as one.

Jouissance, used by Lacan, is a sexual site or sense of incompleteness, so feminine by implication. It locates our futility in another's receptivity. No token feminism, not even female. For the woman is not herself the "site of truth"; she too, writes Lacan, "souls for soul."[20] The oblation of sublation (*Aufhebung*) is not direct insemination—that is "one of those sweet dreams of philosophy"—but seminal semiotics. Each can love the other only in the way each separately faces the knowledge respectively souled for. Each has a relation to the other by relation to a greater unknown. It follows that those who allow themselves to feel the lost object most keenly, those most transcendentally religious, will use language most passionately, "as lovers do." In that way, the projection of ideality, which is that of a coupling otherness, can be the source of health or neurosis, and doubtless why Gillian Rose used carnal love to reclaim a type of spiritual love in *Love's Work*.

This sacramentalizes need-projection, it inverts the Freudian under-world. Freud arrived at the existence of "the unconscious" by retroductive inference from the facts at hand. How else to explain displaced functions—frozen hands, paralyzed limbs—save by the transference from an imperfectly integrated sexuality? Lacan unfroze the libido by word-therapy, so transformed Freud's underworld, the crippling desires arising from a destructive libido. Given the "infinite" play of signifiers found in language—"a carnival of representation"—it must be that language functions like fresh affiliations thrown up from the caldron of the unconscious more than formal chains of inference. Only a deep-seated desire related to the epiphany of the other is able to quell this need. Epiphany, advent, disclosure, enclosure. Little wonder Levinas deflated rationalistic philosophy as never having been able to appreciate the voluptuousness of language. Voluptuousness is a voyeur; its objects are constantly in flight. Here is fission for the soul; nothing by direct infusion of pure Platonic form. With sex, we do more than just put the openings of our excretory and reproductive systems to work for us in gaining pleasure. Desire is, and always remains, insatiable. For Lacan, no such thing as a purely sexual relation exists. Although each partner plays the role of subject to the other's other, this "dispensation," according to Malcolm Bowie,

> can never produce symmetry or reciprocity: language always creates between them an intractable and unsheddable surplus cargo of otherness, a third party ubiquitous and powerful enough to be called [on occasion] God. It is the special virtue of feminine *jouissance* to outplay both these Gods. It is always supplementary to the One and an enemy of any system that may be erected in its honour, and at the same time swoons away from Otherness and its nefarious works.[21]

"Orgasm [Bowie concludes] has seldom been asked to bear a philosophical burden as heavy as this." It is "the one" in search of the many, self-release unto another, the unity which seeks to reunify itself in another. What Freud saw as forced entry, a phallic act, Jung saw as a symbol of wholeness. A mandala is a line of circumscription around a gap, inscription, ingress, cherished congress. For Lacan, the reality of the unconscious is not even a creative ambiguity, as it was for Kierkegaard, it is "lacuna, cut, rupture inscribed in a certain lack."[22] The lack is shown where the text "gapes," where the power of language deconstructs itself.

Can religion live with this warning against object-fulfillment? It helps create it. If the constitutive feature of the unconscious by which Lacan insecures personal identity but resecures desire is demarcated by a lack, it follows that any theology sensitive to Lacanian psycho-linguistics will entail a dynamic iconography of desire. It will be a methodology which interrogates its own desiring structures, represents a flight from truth. The Old Testament warning not to construct false representations is a good example of negative theology deconstructing the gods. Using a variation of Anselm's argument, J. N. Findlay argued that the purest form of theism allows no finite images. Anselm maintained the most perfect conceivable being must necessarily exist—or suffer a blot of imperfection which mars the concept. Findlay reversed it. The most perfect conceivable being must necessarily not exist, or endure a mark of existence which taints the concept with finite imagery. God must, of necessity, transcend all representations absolutely, completely, infinitely. The concept "God" deconstructs itself. In this way, iconoclastic Protestantism, bent on destroying the idols of false representation found in authoritarian religion, is a half-way house to speculative atheism. The purest form of art based on this type of atheology stands farthest from literal truth. Kristeva finds the language of "otherness" reinstated in the image of the Mother and child, in religious iconography. The artistic accomplice of such negative theology is the most creative representations we can find. For Feuerbach, "art is God in the form-determination of sensuous perception."[23] But "God" is also a form determined by the imagination. The art of religion calls for a constant baptism of tongues or gifts of discernment, the spirit of interpretation.

George Steiner employs his version of *via negativa*. "Language is the main instrument of one's refusal to accept the world as it is." Ours is the ability to gainsay or "unsay" the world, "to image and speak it otherwise."[24] The Lacanian ancestry is more patrician than those "logically bastard modes" by which Steiner invites us to go "beyond" language, transcending speech. It is plebeian too. Lacanian semiotics has roots reaching down into the soil of our personal development. For Steiner, "new words are born between the lines." Lacan has shown that the gods, lower case, can be minted from the simulcrum of grammar by negative projection since language is compelled to re-enact conflicts the person cannot resolve interpersonally. That is why life-and-death symbols are often drawn from an acute sense of loss. "Astride the grave the forceps are lovingly applied." In performing his "rechristianization" of Nietzschean nihilism, Cambridge theologian Don Cupitt wrote:

> It is because of all this [the inherent play of the signifier] I see faith not as a privileged way of gaining reassuring supernatural information—as, in short, a superstition—but as an ultimate and creative choice made in a moment of darkness in which all such spurious consolations have been irretrievably lost.[25]

Shades of Nietzsche who said, "We do not get rid of God because we still have faith in grammar." Lacan replied, if we appreciate the alter-other of language, we can still retain an altar of divinity in affectional love. For the place of "the other" is the place of God, hallowed by the sacrament of grace. Grace offers us another as infused presence. Language can become address. God is, on this score, the highest expression of linguistic form. Alterity masks holy otherness.

It is not, accordingly, in the phallic spires reaching heavenward that the mystery of our being resides but in the cavernous vaults of the womb-like chancel which serves to remind us of lost emplacement and the mystification of categories of intellection find preserve in admiration or in adoration. For the object to be found in language is no ordinary object, but a subject who solicits attention and escapes notice at the same time, a subject whose solicitude transcends solitude by invitation of grace. Is it curious that this immediacy should look for symbols of divination in a sublime other? No curiosity at all, given the power of the word to transfix and transform the other. "Adam, where art thou?" by which the cry of the caller merged with the need for response. Writes Buber:

> Man wishes to be confirmed in his being by man and wishes to have a presence in the being of the other. The human person needs confirmation because man as man needs it. An animal does not need to be confirmed, for it is what it is unquestionably. It is different with man. Sent forth from the natural domain of species into the hazard of the solitary category, surrounded by the air of a chaos which came into being with him, secretly and bashfully he watches for a Yes which allows him to be and which can come to him only from one human person to another.[26]

Perhaps that is why the imagination is "the most immediate way of presenting ultimate reality to a human being."[27] For the imagination simultaneously deflects what it affects. And the hiddenness of the sources of joy become that which prompts the language shifter: "the other" in whom we live, move, and have our enlightened linguistic being. *Prosopon,* the many-faced God—self, soul, and social being in one. John Millbank argues that "modern" theology turns on an "exchangist" view of being. Perhaps that is why Bonhoeffer defined Christ as the "man for others," better, "person among others." As Virgil remarked, we make our necessities, as we do our personal reality, by our choice of gods. Such icons of reverence, if properly conceived, host the nurture of others.

Language is so good at covering up its weaknesses, its referential failures and inability to communicate fresh truths, that it requires a subversion from within to redeem itself. Doubtless that is why Paul Ricoeur quipped, "Philosophy was able to survive because of the very banishment of the metaphor."[28] It is suppressed "only" by way of extreme measures. Lacan too called for an apocalypse of metaphors in wrestling with the angel of deliverance. That is why theological methodology is relevant to the Lacanian project. Not only because it offers a litany of inspiration, but because "God-talk" in the absence of a concrete signified is in a unique position to display the active displacement of ordinary signifiers. Theology shifts the focus of language from ontological "cataloguing" to open desire, from pray to play, to quote a free soul of the 1960s. Word-play aligns the dance of the signifiers; it allows us to "celebrate the gay, great happening, illimitably earth."

It has been said poetry refreshes the tongue. Theology in a Lacanian mode defamiliarizes the ordinary. It informs us that nothing is ordinary, everything is (possibly) sublime. Theological language subverts ordinary language by metaphysically subliming the signifiers. It does this from within, no transcendent reference-point "beyond" language is necessary. Theology (remarks Charles Winquist) "has a special role in its capacity to transgress any closure of the symbolic order."[29] It does this by removing the deadly anchor of analyticity. Here is a "nay-saying" which is a "gainsaying." "Desire [Lacan writes] references what discourse is not."[30] And denotation is no destination. We need textual strategies drawn from nurture and solicitation to compensate for our sense of loss, to open up, instead of close down on, truth. No heavy breathing, this is light discourse: Spirit, Dove, and Comforter as one.

Theological discourse, most attuned of all disciplines to the presence of absent signifiers, delimits the impulse to "ground" the signifier in naive realism or transcendent idealism. "For verily our God is a hidden God," saith the Psalmist. Theological discourse instructs that no restricted object for language exists. In looking at the world, we are looking at as many things as we have the capacity to describe. "God" is, on this score, not the instantiation of radical negativity, but the negation of radical instantiation, a *deus absconditus*. "God," the denial of standard reference. In ordinary language, and applied to ordinary language, we don't need lurid descriptions of reality to satisfy predication-principles. The concept "God" functions to unseat or subvert conventional theories of language, to dis-establish the truth-grammarians. Imagine "God," the ultimate subversive; the arch-demythologizer. This concept sees off all other pretenders to the throne. It does so by inviting us to worship at the altar of an unknown Deity. It is as if we have an absent tenant in an open universe. Because it constantly escapes our net of words, this stretches the soul. This "god" invites us to find our form, which is us.

Theology stands at the door and knocks—in defiance of the object. And yet it sublates language. That's why poetry can be generative and theology need not be definitive. In deconstructive hermeneutics, amatory passion and poetry become the "friends" of religion. Love unseats, so unfolds and ingrafts. Why?—because "ingiftedness" is truly exchangist. Here is a cry from the heart which can never fully realize, yet never entirely abandon, the ideal of love. "Eros passion is fled: its twin, the passion of faith, is taunting my head."[31] Contrary to Eliot's "loud lament of the disconsolate chimera," Rose advocates that we need a consoling lament of divine discontent to work out our salvation in this "sin of language and lips," offered as a sacrament of Kierkegaardian fear and trembling. May we ever remain uncontented creatures, baptized in the purgatory of a relentless passion.

For Lacan, desire can neither be disclosed nor fully satiated because it is at the foundation of a consciousness which remains split. As such, unrequited love stands a greater chance of recentring "self" than the Cartesian *cogito*, because, as the loom behind all signifiers, love structures not as an internal subject, but person-to-person, interpersonally. Poetic unction allows us to become, in Peter Abbs' apt phrase, "Addicted to dark, violet, heart-shaped words."[32]

What Lacan did, in effect, was take desire from the dank cellar of Freudian fixation and realign it with the advent of "the other." For him, the "godification" of language represents the search for alterity. Lacan's work has strong links with the negative or apophatic tradition in theology, the dispersal of meaning through the word, first spoken, then heard, finally dissimulated among us. For Freud, the compass still points toward the register of pleasure; for Lacan, the needle hovers on mystery. As with all genuine epiphanies, no person knows the hour of the fulfillment of his or her coveted signifier. We keep our eyes steadily on the hills, from whence cometh our help, but whatever the sound of the last trump; it will not be the sound of a trumpet. We need to loosen up the signifiers. As such, Nietzsche's saying, "We do not get rid of God because we still have faith in grammar," is not so cynical. For the God of grammar is the god of the open signifier. Verbal realists supposed that the order we find in language mirrors a stable order which exists in the world, worse, that the reality of the world presupposes an order that is directly reflected in language. Subject-predicate attribution then mirrors the cynical appointment of tentative nouns and putative objects, that then cast a verificationist wet-blanket on language, testing reference-claims to destruction. But what if the order that exists in language does not work like that? What if language is structured more like the unconscious, with its deeper, darker, preternatural forces of signification stimulated by desire instead of some acid-test of truth? Language can be used not for propositional exactitude or truth rectitude but for petition and exaltation. Once weaned off the pretence of precification, the grammar of assent may allow the ascent of grammar. The sacred can then reoccupy the profane and Spirit can, as Hegel said, gain its truth "by finding itself in absolute dismemberment."

It follows that "only dialogical activity with its delays, anticipations, and waiting, its risks and surprising fulfillments" is capable of this kind of chiliastic expectation, the return of the Spirit, riding on chariots of azure splendor or open texts and tropes of endless meaning. Theological language is full of this drama; of the gods come down to us, to sup with us, walk with us and talk to us, even have sport with us. Philosophy lacks this sense of the mytho-poetic, so it has become arid and unfulfilling. And that is why I have indulged myself in the mirror of your acceptance, putting prismatic images and supplicant models over the reason which sanitizes and fetters.

I review the road we have travelled in a poem:

Language is structured like the unconscious;
    but the unconscious is structured by a lack.
Lack gives rise to desire:
    which desire is, loosely, to matriculate with the (m)other;

But such acts of desiring are stalemated by the imposing presence of the Father;

consciousness becomes split in twain —
into awareness of self and consciousness of the other.
This split-theatre of desire constitutes the very conditions by which consciousness comes
into the world, comes into being;
it co-references self *cum* others; promotes alterity as key to social life.

But the ego of rational adaptation gets in the way of acts of ablation;
we look for symbols of self-transcendence, hunt the world over.
The Christian call is for sacrifice, dispossession of self, loss of pride;
What sets one free is not self-sacrifice or loss of self: —
To give oneself away takes a special talent,
derives from an ingifted "we";
Colloquy it is not flesh seeking incorruption,
but an in-seeking of flesh, allowing otherness.

There is, then, a sureness of self which is always ready to be made unsure
for the sake of others.
It is known as creative insecurity, as faith,
the erotic furnishes us with a prototype of spirit;
it is the basis of our relationship with mystery,
incarnates flesh in order to appropriate others.

There is, then, no purely sexual relation,
because there is no relation that is purely sexual;
it is in the faultlines of communication more than its fitness that
unconscious desire is revealed;
The truth of desire resides in the intersubjective space between self and another.
This space goes unreclaimed by modern philosophy;
literature has put in a bid;
only theology with its negative images and baptism of fire grants us the sphere of the "in-between."

Theology demythologizes the search for truth by deconstructing the philosopher's
lodestone; no holy grail.
But theology also deconstructs its own mythology.
A fortiori, the concept "God" exists not as object, but as desire;
— the soul of desire.

The truth of desire is thus eternal longing,
nay, co-belonging.

As such, we do rush in to fill a space; we do not act in the name of the Father;
we do not display a symbolic phallus full of presence, or plenitude, all-power;
Rather, we matriculate in the image of the Mother, hallowed womb of all becoming.
— hidden place, a secret space
where soul delights to hide;
That hidden disclosure requires a constant emptying of oneself, a sacred carnality.

I can never be finished with emptying of myself from myself;
it is ceaseless redemption;
it is the gnosis of be-coming real in the flesh,
until death us do part.

NOTES

1. Dietrich Bonhoeffer, *Letters and Papers from Prison* (London: SCM Press, 1953), p. 105.

2. Jacques Lacan, *The Four Fundamental Concepts of Psycho-analysis*, trans. Alan Sheridan (New York: Norton, 1978), p. 188; see also Hegel, *The Philosophy of Mind*, trans. William Wallace and A.V. Miller (Oxford: Oxford University Press, 1971), p. 24.

3. Edith Wyschogrod, D. Crownfield, C.A. Raschke, eds., *Lacan and Theological Discourse* (Albany, N.Y.: State University of New York Press, 1989), p. 28.

4. *The Writings of William James, A Comprehensive Edition*, ed. J. McDermott, (New York: Modern Library, 1968), pp. 355-356.

5. Martin Buber, *Eclipse of God*, p. 13.

6. R.D. Laing, *The Divided Self* (New York: Pantheon Books, 1969), pp. 36-37.

7. Jacques Lacan, *The Language of the Self: The Function of Language in Psychoanalysis* (Baltimore: John Hopkins University Press: 1968), p. 57.

8. Peter Abbs, *The Polemics of Imagination* (London: Skoob, 1996), p. 107.

9. Julia Kristeva, *Powers of Horror* (New York: Columbia University Press, 1982), pp. 4, 9.

10. *Ibid.* p. 3.

11. Abbs, *The Polemics of Imagination*, p. 120.

12. Jacques Lacan, *Crits*, ed. Alan Sheridan (New York: Norton, 1977) pp. 119-120.

13. Ibid. p. 86.

14. Lacan, *The Four Fundamental Concepts of Psycho-analysis*, p. 192.

15. Martin Buber, *The Way of Response*, ed. N. N. Glatzer (New York: Schocken Books, 1966), p.108.

16. Gillian Rose, *Love's Work* (New York: Schocken Books, 1995), p. 98.

17. Sean Hand, *The Levinas Reader* (Oxford: Blackwell, 1989), pp. 37, 48, 56 fn. 22, 176, 181.

18. Allen Ginsberg, from "Song," in *Howl and Other Poems* (New York: Harper & Row, 1986).

19. Buber, *The Way of Response*, p. 103.

20. Jacques Lacan, *Feminine Sexuality: Jacques Lacan and the 'Ecole Freudienne,'* selections from Lacan, ed. Mitchell and Rose (London: Macmillan Press, 1982), p. 156.

21. Ibid. p. 154.

22. Lacan, *The Four Fundamental Concepts*, p. 153.

23. Ludwig Feuerbach, *The Principles of the Philosophy of the Future* (Indianapolis: Bobbs-Merrill, 1966), p. 57.

24. See *A Steiner Reader*, p. 398.

25. Don Cupitt, *Modern Theology*, 1:1 (1984), "A Reply to Rowan Williams," pp. 27-28.

26. Buber, *The Way of Response*, p. 208.

27. Peter Abbs, quoting the Welsh poet and parson, R. S. Thomas, *The Polemics of Imagination*, p. 157.

28. Paul Ricoeur, *A Ricoeur Reader*, ed. Mario Valdes (Buffalo: University of Toronto Press, 1991), p. 269.

29. Wyschogrod, Crownfield, Raschke, *Lacan and Theological Discourse*, p. 32.

30. Ibid. p. 30.

31. Rose, *Love's Work*, p. 64.

32. Peter Abbs, "An Undelivered Letter," from *Personae and Other Poems* (London: Skoob, 1995), p. 68.

Five

REDEEMING THE MEMORY OF SUFFERING

Robert N. Fisher

Suffering provokes us to undertake a journey—one which is narrative in character, leading us to an uncompromising and uncharted world of illness, pain, and loss. This journey is prompted by the jarring shock of untamed feelings and untamable passions aroused by the suffering of another human being, be it a friend or a loved one. In the event of the death of someone we cherished, the searing realization of loss penetrates and submerges us again and again, as waves of anguish irrupt over and intrude into our more settled moments. The loss of a person, the sudden absence of a uniquely familiar presence in our lives, the likes of which will never be seen on this planet again, confronts and astounds us. It calls us on a voyage for which we are usually ill-equipped; and we are destined never to set foot on the same shores again. This is a journey which I have come to regard as a passage from a detached view on, to an involved concern with, suffering.

1. Embarking

We cannot escape suffering—that much is sure. When we are confronted face to face with people who are suffering, who are hurting and in pain, we cannot escape asking questions about the "meaning" or the "purpose" of suffering.[1] Why is it that people suffer? Why do those who I care about most, who mean everything to me, suffer anguish and distress? Why should this be? No meaning, reason, or purpose appears to exist.

Yet to ask questions like these reveals that I ask them as an observer; I ask such questions as a spectator—as someone who is detached or removed from the person who is experiencing pain or enduring suffering. I ask it because their suffering induces in, and causes a problem for, me. The question is asked from a detached point of view; it implies an equally detached neutral, generally applicable answer that can be gained independently of the people who are and do suffer. It implies we can arrive at an answer to suffering without having to get involved or dirty our theodical hands in what people are experiencing.

John Hick and Geddes MacGregor make much the same claim: human suffering provokes problems which usually arise "in the mind of the spectator rather than in that of the sufferer."[2] Such suffering becomes the starting point for the voyage which inevitably follows. The suffering observed and witnessed in the course of daily life forms the foundations of Ivan Karamazov's "rebellion"—a rebellion which, out of protest at the suffering caused in him by the reality of suffering seen in the lives of those around him, forces him to "respectfully return" to God his "ticket of admission."[3] After the death of his mother, the doting son in Michael Ignatieff's *Scar Tissue* is left with the problem of finding a way of "redeeming" her memory:

> I still have days when everything she ever was, everything she ever meant to me is entirely erased by the memory of those great agonizing breaths, that frail body wracked with spasms, those lips wet with blood. There must be some way to redeem this, some way to believe that the banal heartlessness of it all was not for nothing.[4]

Having witnessed the prolonged death of a child from plague, both the believing Father Paneloux and the humanist Dr. Rieux are left to grapple with the sense that can be made of the needless suffering of children whose bodies are wasted and destroyed by disease.[5] As Joy Davidman is reported to have said to C.S.Lewis shortly before her own death from cancer, "it is easier for the one who goes first."

What we think we are looking for as we embark on our journey is an answer, a solution that will explain what is happening. We feel that if only we can find the "right" perspective from which to view suffering, then the picture will clarify itself; it will make good sense to us. Yet I suggest that in the first instance, an answer is not what we are looking for. What we want is something that will appease us. The drive to understand is both a coping mechanism to relieve our sense of helplessness, as well as an effort to appease the sense of grievance we feel. Suffering is not just a problem for us; suffering is an outrage to us, something to which we react sharply, which intrudes and affects us at a deeply personal level, at the point where things matter most. We all have something of Ivan inside us; we all feel the sense of injustice, horror, and absurdity when confronted with the suffering of another human being.

But because we are observers indicates two points. First, it reveals something about the nature of suffering and pain. Second, it reveals something about the way we relate to suffering and pain. The first thing it reveals is that suffering and pain are never directly present to us. Suffering is invisible. As I write these words, I am in pain. Across the room my wife knows nothing of the draining, ever present nagging that is the horizon within which I live and work. At best, she infers it—from a grimace when I move, from the slow and awkward way I change position as I sit at the desk. We never see pain directly; we never have direct and immediate access to it. A way of objectively measuring pain, or forming criteria by means of which a person's suffering can be assessed can never exist. Pain is always their pain, suffering will always be their individual suffering—unique to them. However, that pain and suffering, because it lies hidden "below the surface," is easily susceptible of being ignored or not believed.

What is easy to do, and what is equally hurtful and wrong, is to move from thinking that because pain cannot be seen, it does not therefore exist. A person can suffer without carrying the visible signs of anguish. But such suffering can be heightened, and the anguish made sharper by not being believed.

Suffering is unique—is always my suffering, uniquely personal and private to me. No matter how much I feel for another person or empathize for the anguish suffered by another person, I cannot enter into that suffering, nor can I experience the other person's pain. Only I know what it means for me to suffer or be in pain. This is why pain and suffering is a problem to the observer. In relation to another person's suffering, no one is in any kind of position to evaluate pain in a meaningful or final way. Just because suffering is so private, so intimately connected with the personal experience and history of the individual, we are compelled to agnosticism about its "worth" or "meaning."

We might want to say that a person's suffering is "evil"; but such a judgment is based on my imaginative response to what it would be like for me to experience and suffer that pain. This is precisely what we cannot do. Although the physical quality of the pain might be the same, its personal meaning and effects are not. I am in no position to say whether your experience will prove to be of any value or worth, either in itself or in the long term. I can sympathize with you; I can offer you support and comfort during the experience. But I am compelled to be agnostic as to whether it may prove to be of "worth" within your life history.

These considerations point to a second feature of pain and suffering, namely, that it defies even the usual kinds of meaning and explanation people try to make of or place on suffering. As something uniquely intimate to the experience and history of the individual, even those closest to the sufferer, who love the sufferer, cannot chart the way it invades, develops within, and affects the life of the person loved. A barrier between sufferer and carer exists; the carer cannot possibly "share" in the experience of the sufferer.

The barrier is exacerbated because the sufferer has no way of communicating objectively the meaning of his or her pain. Even language ruptures and implodes under the weight of pain. Suffering defies language and evades all attempts at expression. At best, it can capture the surface of pain, or fix on and describe a fleeting quality.[6] But that is not the pain. Tolstoy captures the sense well. Having been badgered into taking the final sacrament by a wife who does not understand, nor even attempts to understand the depths of his torment, Ivan Ilyich is enticed into admitting for the sake of those present that he feels better:

> And as soon as he admitted that thought his exasperation returned and with it the agonizing physical suffering and with the suffering a consciousness of the unavoidable, approaching end. To this was added a new sensation of grinding shooting pain and a feeling of suffocation. The expression on

> his face when he uttered that 'Yes' was dreadful. Having pronounced it he looked at her straight in the eye, turned on his face with a rapidity extraordinary in his weak state and shouted: 'Go away, go away. Leave me alone!'
> From that moment the screaming began that continued for three days and was so awful that one could not hear it through closed doors two rooms away without horror. At the moment when he answered his wife he realized that he was lost, that there was no return, that the end had come, the very end, while his doubts were still unsolved and remained doubt.
> 'Oh! Oh! Oh!' he cried in varying intonations.[7]

We hear in Tolstoy the real language of pain—expressed in whimpers, shrieks, cries, screams, and tears. This "pre-language" or "sub-language" demonstrates that suffering "shatters" language and destroys the world which language has constructed for our lives.[8]

Suffering is met with a desire to search for meaning and articulate what is being endured. The desire forces the experience of pain into language—into the public "objective" space that exists between people. But when the climax or wave of pain overcomes the sufferer again, language breaks down, shatters, and we revert again to cries and groans. Like a tide that moves in and out, so pain and language share the same relationship. The sufferer tries desperately to get a handle on the suffering, tries to speak of it and rationalize it—to get it "out there" in the objective public world for all to see, understand, and share. But then the tide comes in, and the person slips back into the only means of communication they have—screams, tears, and the contorted, awkward movements of the body in pain. This, if anything, is the language of suffering.

However, if suffering is unique and if pain has no language, how can we do theodicy? How can we search for explanations, answers, and solutions? What can be said in the presence of those who are hurting? No coherent system of explanation, no set of values or beliefs can apparently be placed on, or arise out of suffering. Suffering and pain fundamentally undermine all our usual ways of explaining and making sense of things. Suffering affects everything, nothing we think, believe, or value, remains untouched and unaffected by the experience of suffering. Suffering affects, influences, and colors everything. It becomes the horizon against which our lives are lived.

On the face of it, to try to talk about suffering is futile. When you are face to face with someone who is screaming in pain, or enduring constant, nagging suffering from which they can gain little or no relief, what is farcical is the attempt to try and justify or explain what is happening to them. In the presence of suffering our whole being should protest, should feel revulsion at the attempt to justify. What can be said to a mother who has just lost her six-month old daughter? What can be said to the husband who has seen his wife of forty years gradually degenerate, ravaged with rheumatoid arthritis, every movement of her body accompanied by excruciating pain? What do you say?

I want to propose that you say nothing. You say nothing because nothing needs to be said. For once we must learn to shut up, and to acquire the delicate art of silence which signifies your patient "being there" for the sufferer. Absolutely nothing can ever do away with the pain and hurt someone goes through. Nothing can "redeem" chronic pain—its violence, ferocity, and sheer random absurdity. Nor can the memory of such pain be magically erased, or made "alright," or subsumed into an explanation which will make sense of it all.

2. The Voyage

I do not, however, advocate the idea that we should not try to speak of suffering. I do not want to say we should not try to seek the meaning of suffering, if any meaning exists. Instead, I sound the cautious note that if such an attempt is made, then we need to have a sharply focused idea of what is being aimed at, and to whom it will be aimed. What is frighteningly easy is to sit and "do" theodicy in a context removed from and which pays little heed to the voices of those who suffer. Such theodicies have a habit of sounding either alien or crassly insensitive when transposed into the context of the sufferer.

We might wonder to whom Farrer would address the following words: "If what we say is neither comforting nor tactful, we need not mind. Our business is to say, if we can, what is true."[9] The implicit hint here is that what is suffered and what is true are not one and the same thing. Indeed, Farrer admits the distinction by claiming "so far from beginning with the sufferer and his personal distresses, we will attempt to get the issue into perspective."[10] Again, the implicit principle at work appears to be that when the sufferer's personal distress is put "into perspective" then it will be seen for what it "really" is, that is, not suffering, or not as "dark" an episode in the person's life as it initially appears.[11]

The attitude of detachment seemingly imposed on the observer of suffering (and prized by the theodicist) is mistaken. It may be that those who either "intentionally or inadvertently" construct responses which "occlude the radical and ruthless particularity of human evil" do mediate a "social and political practice which averts its gaze from the cruelties that exist in the world."[12] But such a response fails to notice a second set of issues associated with the fact of our being observers of suffering, namely, what it tells us about the way we relate to suffering and pain.

For while we are primarily observers of suffering and pain, we are never detached observers. To speak of suffering, or to even raise the questions prompted by suffering in the first place, is to be witness to your own relation to suffering. In other words, we cannot speak of suffering without bringing ourselves and our experiences into the picture as well. When you speak of suffering, you speak of the experiences and feelings which lead you into asking the question about suffering. One sufferer never exists—always two, because suffering is inter-personal.

I joke that when my wife gave birth to our first child, I had a worse labor and delivery than she did! The pain was intense, long and protracted, and my sense of frustration at the inability to do anything to help her when it became too much that she had to cry out and scream only served to heighten and mock my impotence to alleviate in any way the suffering of the person I love. For Fiona, the pain of labor was ultimately an intensely creative experience—and that is why, for her, the suffering endured is a distant memory. But the pain of my own helplessness in the presence of her screams still haunts and taunts me. The suffering of those with terminal illness is destructive—not creative; and the suffering of those who love them is unbearable in its impotence.

The point is made by Gabriel Marcel:

> I can only grasp something as evil in the measure in which it touches me—that is to say, in the measure in which I am involved, as one is involved in a lawsuit. Being 'involved' is the fundamental fact; I cannot leave it out of account except by an unjustifiable fiction, for in doing so, I proceed as though I were God, and a God who is an onlooker at that.[13]

The "problem" of suffering naturally arises in the mind of the spectator rather than that of the sufferer. The sufferer's immediate task is to face and cope with the pain being experienced and endured. Those who suffer do not want or need someone around "doing" theodicy; what they need is practical assistance in their enduring—the offer of hope, the holding of a hand, a reassuring smile. For them, suffering is not a riddle to be solved, but is something to be born and lived through.

Those who ask the question of suffering do so as people who suffer for them. Their suffering prompts in us suffering; the wanting to reach out, yet the sense of helplessness, the anger, frustration, and hopelessness of not being able to do anything to relieve the suffering of the one we love. That hurts—so much.

What it also brings is the start of the transition from a detached to an involved view of suffering. The psychological process is captured perfectly by Tolstoy. On the death of Ivan Ilyich, Piotr Ivanovich visits the widow, where they politely discuss Ivan's last hours:

> The thought of the sufferings of the man he had known so intimately, first as a light-hearted child, then a youngster at school, and later on, when they were grown up, as a partner at whist, suddenly struck Piotr Ivanovich with horror....
>
> 'Three days and nights of awful suffering and then death. Why, it might happen to me, all of a sudden, at any moment,' he thought, and for an instant he was terrified. But immediately, he could not have explained how,

> there came to his support the old reflection that this thing had befallen Ivan Ilyich and not him, and that it ought not and could not happen to him, and that to think that it could meant that he was falling into a melancholy frame of mind, which was a mistake... After which reflection Piotr Ivanovich cheered up and began to ask with interest about the details of Ivan Ilyich's end, as though death were some mischance to which only Ivan Ilyich was liable, but he himself was not.[14]

We glimpse in Piotr Ivanovich the clash and sudden but momentary collapse of the detached perspective into an involved perspective—when a person leaves a state of detachment and is drawn into a more personal and involved relationship with suffering. It draws us closer and starts the processes of thought about our own suffering, even our own eventual death because this is the suffering of someone we know, or love. But that happens just for a while. A small chink in our armour appears against which the detachment of the observer's position serves as a protective mechanism and which instantly deflects our attention away.

The closer the person suffering is to us, the more it "hits home" as the suddenness of the collapse of one perspective into the other occurs, and the more deeply it hurts. The clash of these two perspectives is seen when the doctor and the son of an ailing mother in *Scar Tissue* discuss her condition:

> The doctor looks at Mother's....scans and sees a disease of memory function, with a stable name and a clear prognosis. I see an illness of selfhood, without a name or even a clear cause.[15]

The people who care for those undergoing hospital treatment, clinical surgery, or any kind of medical assessment stand on the front line where these perspectives clash. They may seek to understand the condition, treatment, and fate of the person they love. To do this, they must rise to the level of detached objectivity in which the language used by doctors to describe the present state of the patient is couched. Or these words have to be transposed into the context of the intimate and deeply personal relationship they share with the sufferer, the implications it has not just for the sufferer but for themselves as well. The transition between or collapse of the two perspectives arises from the context of our interpersonal relationships—from the people we care about, and those whom we love. Their suffering draws us to them; it forces us to contemplate our own eventual suffering, and demise. And the more we care, the more we love, the more profoundly it will draw us in, the more deeply it will engage us.

3. Disembarking

Can anything be said from an involved perspective? Perhaps—but I am not sure what, and I'm not sure I have the words to do it justice. But I must try. The son's words from *Scar Tissue*, on discovering that he also has the initial tell-tale signs of Alzheimer's disease, serve as a good starting point:

> I long to know, to be certain, to be face to face with the thing itself. I long to be able to see the pathways of my own brain. My brother is right. No antidote to fear compares with knowledge.
>
> The brew that is true is bubbling away in the chalice with the palace. Soon it will be approved and prescribed, to arrest the pathological cascade, and in the standard scientific manner, to transform fate into a condition, to convert tragedy into something ordinary and unremarkable. As Kafka says, there is hope, but not for us. It will come too late for me.
>
> I want to predict it in every particular. I want to imagine it as far as I can. What else is the examined life for? Is the manner in which I have come to understand it going to alter the way it takes me over? Is a disease observed altered by the attempt to observe it?
>
> It is not as far-fetched a thought. Everybody goes through it differently. No one is ever just a case, a pure instance of the condition. A certain margin of individuality is allowed to each of us.... Everyone finds their own path to extinction.[16]

The son's reaction is touchingly illuminating—and, I think, invites us to travel a difficult path.

The first stage of the path is the removal of unnecessary suffering and fear by becoming acquainted with the facts—to try and demystify the processes that are at work when a person suffers, or is in the final stages of life. Hiding the facts from the sufferer, although well intentioned, removes the possibility of not only understanding the nature of the situation, but of acting and achieving something, anything, in the light of that knowledge. A strange comfort and security can be had from such knowledge. It can help us to anticipate, and even direct, the course of our going.

The problem is that so often, and far too easily, the sufferer surrenders control of their illness and themselves, on entering hospital or in giving themselves over to the care of the local doctor and family. Illness belongs to patients—not persons. We give up control to other people; and the one thing that made us peculiarly us—our agency, our ability to interact responsively with others—becomes the first casualty. We are, quite voluntarily and almost pathetically, robbed of the major tool which fashions personal identity. And to give it up is to give up our humanity and our personality. We become the depersonalized patients of a diagnosed condition, prescribed by those who know us not. And as objects of care, we become less than the persons we are in the eyes of family and friends. Suffering, like treatment and care, is something we passively undergo.

To know of someone's condition is a form of control over the situation, and a refusal to let go of the interpersonal character of what is, or what should be happening, and a demand to be treated as such. "Nothing could be more beautiful than to see it happen: the molecular progress of your own dying."[17] It may offer us the opportunity to compose in our minds or anticipate the way in which we will bring down the curtain on our own life on earth. We want a peaceful death; we want to die well—for our own sake, and for the sake of those who will be with us in our final moments. We almost expect to die well—to die with dignity.

Yet expectations rarely match up with what happens. The end of life can either be brutally abrupt or else chart a course through a series of degenerative and painful events that involve the break-down and disintegration of the person and the person's humanity. The question of dignity may not even arise.[18] And if we are asking about the "meaning" of suffering, or of redeeming the suffering of those we love, or of our own suffering, what can be said?

Quite simply this: our hope of redemption lies in the meaning of what our lives have been. The son in *Scar Tissue* does not want to be "eternally condemned to think of her as she was in those final moments, when we held her hands, my brother and I, and she fought for life and lost, her mouth stretched open, gasping for breath, her eyes staring sightlessly up into the lights." This is precisely the suffering and the memory of suffering, that must be redeemed. He wants to remember her as she was; "that is how she should be remembered. That is what I must rescue from her dying, if such a thing can be done."[19] Redemption lies in finding the memory of what a person meant—both to themselves as well as for us. Immediately after her death, C. S .Lewis always complained he could not remember Joy's face; yet he redeemed the memory of her suffering by rediscovering the meaning of her life, and the nature of the relationship they shared. Hope resides in the meaning of what our lives have been—and what they can be.

On this basis alone we can say two things. First, we must attempt to make suffering, even death, an interpersonal experience. At the most fundamental level, this means we must not let a person suffer and die in isolation—in a state alien to their existence as a person. It represents Ivan Ilyich's single, most overwhelming dread:

> Of late, in the loneliness in which he found himself, lying with his face to the back of the sofa, a loneliness in the midst of a populous town and surrounded by numerous acquaintances and relations—loneliness more complete than could be found anywhere, be it at the bottom of the sea or

> in the bowels of the earth—of late in this fearful loneliness Ivan Ilyich had lived only in memories of the past.[20]

To be alone in pain; to be isolated in your suffering, to have no one to reach out to, or to love and be loved by, ruthlessly truncates all sense of being a person and increases and intensifies suffering. It is to be ignored when we yearn to be noticed most: "the most wretched thing of all for Ivan Ilyich was that nobody pitied him as he yearned to be pitied. At certain moments, after a prolonged bout of suffering, he craved more than anything—ashamed as he would have been to own it—for someone to feel sorry for him as if he were a sick child."[21]

Death, dying, and suffering, are intersubjective acts—acts we have to share with those who love us. We must be allowed to die or to suffer with each other, in the company and companionship of those who love us. It makes a difference to our suffering; it can make the world of difference to our ending. Being inter-subjective and interpersonal, the event is one which involves all of us, and so is colored and shaped by those who are present.

But such a consideration only makes imperative the second thing we need to attempt to do; that is, the attempt to let go and let be. At a practical level, for example, this means we should avoid prolonging unnecessary treatments—avoid trying to snatch or beg for that extra five or ten minutes more life for those we love—or even extra days. This is too often a huge disservice to those whom we love—and it represents our forceful domination over someone else's pain and suffering. To wish so stringently and so urgently for extra time, though natural, ignores the interpersonal character of what is happening, and accentuates our own desires and wishes. A time will come when those extra snatched moments at the end of a life are not worth the additional suffering it brings to the person, and the lingering it forces. We must recognize their personhood; their right to say goodbye when they are ready. We must allow people to die; we must say to them, and tell them, "it is all right to die." We must let go.

These are indeed foreign shores. They are shores where the meaning of hope is still being forged, and is forged anew each time we are brought to them. I live with the hope that the meaning I strive to create in my life, the way that I live, the relationships I form, the bonds that somehow tie people together, will be the memory that people redeem from my passing away; it will be the memory and appreciation of my person. The meaning of my life will be something which emerges because it flowed through a life lived to the full, enjoyed, savored, appreciated for the opportunities it has brought my way, and a thankfulness that I have been given the chance. I have no regrets.

I want to be allowed to go in my own way, with those whom I love and who love me. People will find hope in their faith in God; that is fine. People will want to achieve one last thing: that too, is their hope. Whatever it may be, each of us must find hope in his or her own way. And each of us must learn to love in his or her own way, a love which lets go, which values and affirms the worth of what has been. Persons are unique, and unrepeatable. The death of the person is the death of something never seen again. The loosing, the vanishing of people we love, forever, is not an easy thing to continue to live with. But we can give their lives and their dying meaning by letting go—letting go because of what the person has meant to us, and because we love that person for the memory of what he or she continues to mean to us. That is the hope we can give to the suffering of those we love. This is a way of redeeming suffering.

NOTES

1. Frances Young, *Face to Face* (London: Epworth Press, 1985).

2. John Hick, *Evil and the God of Love*, Fontana Library Theology and Philosophy, 2nd impression (London: Macmillan, 1970), p. 10. Geddes MacGregor, *An Introduction to Religious Philosophy* (Boston: Houghton Mifflin Co., 1959), pp. 331-332.

3. Fyodor Dostoyevsky, *The Brothers Karamazov*, translated by D. Magarshack, 2 Vols. (Harmondsworth, Middlesex: Penguin Books, 1978), Vol. 1, p. 286.

4. Michael Ignatieff, *Scar Tissue: A Novel* (London: Chatto and Windus, 1993), p. 1.

5. Albert Camus, *The Plague*, translated by S. Gilbert (Harmondsworth, Middlesex: Penguin Books, 1985), p. 178.

6. See Ronald Melzack and Patrick Wall, *The Challenge of Pain* (Harmondsworth, Middlesex, Penguin Books, revised ed., 1991), ch. 1, part 3, "The Varieties of Pain."

7. Leo Tolstoy, *The Death of Ivan Ilyich and Other Stories*, translated by R. Edmonds (Harmondsworth, Middlesex: Penguin Books, 1960), pp. 158-159.

8. See Elaine Scarry, *The Body in Pain: The Making and Unmaking of the World* (Oxford: Oxford University Press, 1985).

9. Austin Farrer, *Love Almighty and Ills Unlimited*, The Fontana Library of Theology and Philosophy (London: Collins, 1966), p. 7.

10. *Ibid.*

11. Terrence Tilley, *The Evils of Theodicy* (Washington: Georgetown University Press, 1990), ch. 9.

12. Kenneth Surin, *Theology and the Problem of Evil* (Oxford: Basil Blackwell, 1986), p. 51.

13. Gabriel Marcel, *The Philosophy of Existence*, translated by Manya Harari, The Changing World Series (London: Harvill Press, 1948), p. 9.

14. Tolstoy, *The Death of Ivan Ilyich*, pp. 107-108.

15. Michael Ignatieff, *Scar Tissue*, p. 60.

16. *Ibid.*, p. 198.

17. *Ibid.*, p. 194.

18. See Sherwin Nuland, *How We Die: Reflections on Life's Final Chapter* (New York: A. A. Knopf, 1994).

19. Ignatieff, *Scar Tissue*, p. 1.

20. Tolstoy, *The Death of Ivan Ilyich*, pp. 154-155.

21. *Ibid.*, pp. 143-144.

Six

THE DIALECTICS OF DISTANCE AND DEPENDENCE

Patricia Sayre and Linnea Vacca

Endlessly imaginative, most playful when most metaphysical, Luigi Pirandello's works raise serious questions about the sticky problems we encounter in trying to understand personhood. A distinctive characteristic of persons is their ability to view the world at some distance from their own immediate concerns. But while some ways of getting distance from our lives can lead to a more humane apprehension of ourselves and others, other forms of distancing have monstrous potentials. In the first section of our chapter, we draw on a limited selection of Pirandello's works to illustrate the ways self-protective distancing can set up morally problematic matrices of dependence between persons. In the second section, we return to those same works to find hints of a more self-aware mode of distancing that can serve to transform the potentially monstrous into the humane. Although self-aware distancing has its risks, we suggest that it also has a critical contribution to make to our ability to respond compassionately to other persons.

1.

Pirandello's short story, "A Character's Tragedy," opens with the first-person narrator describing his "old habit of giving audience every Sunday morning to the characters of [his] future short stories."[1] Into this audience one week intrudes Dr. Fileno, the creation of another writer. Fileno is the only personage with any vivacity in an otherwise moribund novel. He wants the narrator of Pirandello's story, intended to represent Pirandello himself, to rescue him from the world created by his original, mediocre author, and to provide him with a more adequate setting for his development as a character. Dr. Fileno wants to become the character he feels he truly ought to be so that the world can profit from his life's work, *The Philosophy of Distance*. This mammoth but not yet published book describes a method by which humankind can be cured of all its ills. The method is to read history books "from morning till night" to become adept at "looking on the present as history too—that is, as something already very remote in time."[2] By placing himself in the future to look back at a present he views as already the past, Dr. Fileno can find consolation for every calamity, including the loss of a child. When a friend visits to commiserate with Fileno a few days after his daughter's death, he finds that Fileno has no need of his condolences; from Fileno's perspective, the death is as though it had occurred centuries ago. The impersonal consolation supplied by his philosophy has eliminated any need for the personal activity of consoling.

In its intentions, Fileno's method is humane. Based on a tacit acknowledgment that we can know what others feel and suffer, it compassionately promises to reduce the horrible pain of living to "an austere, serene peace, permeated with that certain sadness without regret which the cemeteries on the earth's surface would still retain even after all the people on earth had died out."[3] This philosophy fosters a compassion so cosmic that it can exist independently of living human beings. And yet how monstrous that a father should feel so little grief on the death of his daughter. Monstrous, but not surprising. To the extent that Fileno succeeds in living in accord with his philosophical outlook, he becomes almost by definition incapable of mourning the passing of his child. In his affective independence from the world, he has withdrawn from the flesh and blood presence of his daughter long before her death was even an issue.

Cultivating a philosophical distance that leaves persons as good as alone in the world is a project not unique to Dr. Fileno. The historical remotion he employs has an epistemological counterpart in the solipsistic starting point bequeathed to modern thought by Descartes. Even if few of us are inclined seriously to doubt the existence of other people, Cartesian methodology involves a remotion from our ordinary lived experience that raises serious doubts about our ability to know what other people are thinking and feeling. These doubts are explored in some detail in another Pirandello work, the play *It* Is *So! (If You Think So).*

The action opens with the leading citizens of a provincial town in an uproar over the strange behavior of a newcomer, Signor Ponza. Ponza has rented a flat for his mother-in-law across town from the flat he rents for his wife and himself. Rumor has it that he keeps his wife locked up and allows her mother to see her "only from a distance."[4] As the townspeople devise schemes to uncover the reason for these peculiar family relations, Laudisi (the character who comes closest to speaking for Pirandello himself) tells them that their curiosity is useless: "What can we really know about other people—who they are—what they are—what they are doing, and why they are doing it?"[5] He himself, he is sure, is a different person to everyone he encounters, and any attempt others might make to get at the "real truth" about him is bound to fail.

The townspeople's immediate response to Laudisi's skepticism is to dismiss it on the grounds that an easy way to find the truth about others exists: ask them. In the case of Signor Ponza and his family, however, employing this strategy only makes matters worse. Ponza claims that his mother-in-law, Signora Frola, is mad and is being kept at a distance from his wife because his wife is not her daughter. Her daughter died four years ago, and Ponza's wife is his second wife. When his first wife died, Signora Frola suffered a complete mental break down. At the time of his second marriage, however, she recovered her sanity in every regard but one: she believes his second wife to be her daughter, who had not died. Ponza, concerned to prevent another break down, supports her in this delusion—which necessitates keeping her at some distance from his wife. Signora Frola, for her part, claims that four years ago Ponza went mad; her daughter was taken from him for a time, and when she returned he was convinced that she was another woman. A mock remarriage was arranged, and since that time, Signora Frola has supported Ponza in his delusion, for he is apparently sane in all other regards—a good man who makes her daughter happy. Both stories fit the evidence, yet both cannot be true.

The difficulties associated with finding the real truth about another person have an analog, Pirandello suggests, in difficulties associated with trying to find the real truth about oneself. Addressing himself before the mirror Laudisi raises the same quandaries the townspeople face in the case of Ponza and his mother-in-law:

> LAUDISI: So there you are! [*He bows to himself and salutes, touching his forehead with his fingers.*] I say, old man, who is mad, you or I? [*He levels a finger menacingly at his image in the glass; and, of course, the image in turn levels a finger at him. As he smiles, his image smiles.*] Of course, I understand! I say it's you, and you say it's me. You—you are mad! No? It's me? Very well! It's me! Have it your way. Between you and me, we get along very well, don't we! But the trouble is, others don't think of you just as I do; and that being the case, old man, what a fix you're in![6]

The "fix" is one common to us all whenever we try to understand ourselves. We assume that in our own case, we know exactly what we are thinking and feeling, and that we are consequently privy to the real truth about why we behave as we do. But are we? How can we be sure that the curiosity with which we approach ourselves, trying to discover the reasons for our own behavior, is not every bit as useless as the curiosity the townspeople direct toward Ponza and his family? We devise explanations for our actions by appeal to underlying mental states to which we assume we have a privileged access. But can we be sure that we are not supporting ourselves in delusions we have devised in order to keep ourselves from confronting a real truth that would leave us devastated? Perhaps we are all the victims of a partial madness that is our only protection from complete insanity.

To return to Dr. Fileno, we can see that he is, if not mad, then engaged in serious self-delusion. While Dr. Fileno might present himself to Pirandello as a great philosopher, he is just someone else's character, an escapee from a bad novel, trying to persuade Pirandello to make him his so that his method can be disseminated as it deserves. But hold on, he already is Pirandello's character! No evidence supports that this alleged bad novel is anything but a fiction in Pirandello's story.

These are clever and playful contradictions; underneath, however, is a serious one. Compare Fileno's avowed method of distancing with his behavior in the story—his urgent, increasingly strident efforts to get Pirandello to adopt him. Dr. Fileno's felt need for another creator shows that he is unable by himself to sustain the stoic independence of persons and circumstance that his philosophy of distance requires. Yet, instead of throwing his method into doubt by acknowledging his dependence on factors and persons lying outside his control, Fileno chooses to hold on to the method, attempting to extend the field of his control by bullying a new author into developing him as he, Fileno, thinks he should be developed. And so Dr. Fileno manifests yet another form of distancing with monstrous potentials: a distancing of oneself from oneself that makes it impossible to see the contradiction between a philosophical view and the way it has been promulgated—a form of self-delusion that contains the seeds of tyranny.

The connection between distance, self-delusion, and tyranny is played out in a variety of ways in Pirandello's stories. In offering his philosophy of distance to the world, Fileno assumes not only the generality of the problem of human suffering—other people must feel pain, as I do—but also the generality of his solution: other people, feeling what I feel, will want to put those strong painful feelings far away. Never once does it occur to him that other human beings may prefer to experience pain if that is the cost of a life rich in human feeling. In this regard, he resembles elderly Professor Toti in the story "Think It Over, Giacomino!" Professor Toti is well disposed toward his young wife, Maddalena, whose marriage to him brought her financial security and a modest degree of social status. Toti has manipulated—coerced would not be too strong a word—one of his previous students into becoming the "secret" lover by whom Maddalena has had a child. Aware that he is not an attractive spouse, Toti is sure that Maddalena could not possibly love him for himself, so he has made suitable arrangements for her. When Toti comes into a considerable fortune, however, he is mildly regretful that it had not come his way earlier. As a rich man he would not have had to make all those alternative arrangements: sharing his wealth would have been recompense enough for having married him. But things are as he has arranged them, and a young wife should be grateful to a husband who supplies her with all she (presumably) wants: a comfortable home, a vigorous lover, a charming toddler. Indeed, at first everyone is pleased by the arrangement. When it begins to disintegrate, Toti cannot fathom why the young man, Giacomino, would want to become engaged to another young woman, brutally abandoning his beloved and his son.

Toti prides himself on being self-aware: "He's a philosopher."[7] He knows what he is doing in orchestrating his wife and her lover's lives, and he knows why he is doing it. The presumption is that Toti has a far wider perspective on the situation than either Maddalena or Giacomino. But somewhere along the way in his arrangements, recognition of Maddalena's and Giacomino's (and his) humanity has been lost. Like an author writing a novel, Toti has created a storied life for his wife and her lover; their roles are to be characters in a narrative line of Toti's own construction. But while Toti, as narrator, appears to dwell cosmically above the worries and fears of the world of real human emotions, his behavior when the story he has constructed goes awry tells a different tale—the tale of a man deeply afraid of being hurt by those around him. The perplexity and agitation he feels as things start to go wrong are inexplicable to him just because he has so completely removed himself from the feelings motivating his manipulations; knowing the logical reasons for these manipulations helps not a wit.

In turning others' lives into a satisfying narrative that he can control, Toti exhibits a remotion similar to Dr. Fileno's. Such remotion is implicit in acts of narration—and not only in the historical narratives of which Fileno is so fond, but also in the professional act of writing a character's story, as well as in our everyday habit of telling our own as well as others' stories. As story-tellers, we step outside the story to adopt a distanced perspective that includes but is not included within the perspectives of others. In this way, we find it natural to assume, either knowingly or unknowingly, that our own perspectives are superior to the perspectives of those whose stories we tell. This assumption is made by the townspeople in *It* Is *So! (If You Think So)* as they attempt to concoct a story that will get at the "real truth" about Signor Ponza and Signora Frola. Standing outside and above the peculiar domestic arrangements about which they have been given such contradictory accounts, they are convinced that their benevolent duty is to construct a coherent account to settle the matter of who is mad. In the process, they force Ponza and his mother-in-law to undergo a series of interviews eventually devolving into something that, as Ponza puts it, "is just plain persecution, plain persecution!"[8] To make matters worse, although the townspeople know that the reason the newcomers have come to their town is the recent devastation of their village in an earthquake that left all their relatives dead, little compassion is shown regarding this circumstance, as the business of producing a coherent narrative about the identity of Ponza's wife swiftly becomes the matter of paramount importance.

Distancing, then, is a practice we find not only in the philosophical methodology put forward by Dr. Fileno as the "philosophy of distance," or in the epistemological counterpart to his historical remotion that we find in the abstract theorizing characteristic of much modern philosophy, but also in the storytelling that is part of our everyday life. And, even when we are careful, we may still find that our capability to assume a distanced perspective on our affairs has blinded us to the reality of other persons, either causing them to vanish from our world, or so imprisoning them in our versions of their story. When they finally do break free from our tyrannical benevolence, we discover that the cost in pain and suffering is monstrously high.

2.

Edwin Arlington Robinson's poem, "Eros Turannos," speaks of the power of town gossip to impose its own interpretations on the lived reality of other human beings.[9] Robinson's persona concludes that this sort of narrative imposition, although most likely erroneous, "does no harm." But in the Pirandello texts we have seen, and in our ordinary lives, we see that it often does a great deal of harm in its denial of full personhood to those who become characters in the narration. And yet, while Pirandello is fascinated with the monstrous potentials inherent in narrative and other forms of distancing, each of the works discussed in the previous section also contains hints of more humane potentials.

In "Think It Over, Giacomino!" these hints are admittedly faint. Given the self-delusion inherent in Professor Toti's situation, it comes as no surprise that the benevolence motivating his tyranny, while real enough, is extremely shallow. Indeed, it disappears altogether once the situation no longer is fully under his control. Learning of Giacomino's plans to marry, Toti goes in the space of minutes from tearful remorse to shouted threats to see to it that Giacomino lose his job. Worse yet, Toti's demeanor toward the child shifts swiftly from impassioned embraces to a willingness to undo Giacomino by showing up at his fiancee's house hand in hand with the little one. The most we can say to redeem this situation is that nothing in Pirandello's telling of Toti's story suggests that it had to take the nasty turn it did. What is possible is that, instead of heightening his mania for narrative control, the confrontation with Giacomino might have awakened in Toti an appreciation of not being the only one with a story to tell—indeed, our awareness of this missed opportunity is precisely what makes "Think It Over, Giacomino!" such a tragedy.

The townspeople in *It* Is *So! (If You Think So)*, like Professor Toti, are after a narrative control subordinating the contradictory perspectives of others to their own hopefully more coherent one. Unlike Toti, however, they are in the process of constructing a narrative instead of trying to maintain their hold on a narrative that has already been constructed. Thus room exists for a voice—Laudisi's—to speak against the wisdom of pushing on with their inquiries. Throughout the play, Laudisi resolutely refuses to speculate on the "real story" the townspeople so greedily pursue. He tries hard to undermine the gossips' "truth seeking" by showing how riddled with uncertainty their project must be. Despite his efforts, the townspeople can rein in neither their curiosity nor the monstrously insensitive behavior to which it gives rise. In the end, the pressure of town gossip virtually subpoenas the woman on whose identity narrative coherence depends. She is the current wife of Signor Ponza. But is she his first and only wife, in which case she is also Signora Frola's daughter, and

Signor Ponza must be mad? Or is she his second wife, in which case she is not Signora Frola's daughter and so the poor Signora must be mad? Signora Ponza's response: "The truth? Simply this: I am the daughter of Signora Frola...and the second wife of Signor Ponza...and, for myself, I am nobody!...I am who you believe me to be!" The play concludes with Laudisi's laughter: "And there, my friends, you have the truth!"[10]

As is almost always the case with Pirandello, the story is more involved than it first appears. Although the story line ends in contradiction, in its emotional weight his play presents the case for compassionate understanding over narrative control. Unexpectedly, the capability of human persons to forge compassionate bonds between themselves, even in the face of the irreconcilability of their stories, wins the day. Although we are left hanging as to what "really" happened between the members of this unusual family before their move into town, the closing scenes of the play leave little doubt that they will continue their efforts to sustain a decent human life for each other, supporting one another in what each considers a delusion. Signora Frola, Signor Ponza, and Signora Ponza, unlike Professor Toti, are not tragic figures for they have discovered something he has not. Willingness to abandon control and allow other stories to stand even when they contradict our own can, on some occasions, create a space for genuine compassion to emerge.

In *It* Is *So! (If You Think So)*, Pirandello shows by example how significant compassion is. In "A Character's Tragedy," he explicitly asserts that although it would take a sympathetic critic to see it, he writes with great compassion for his characters.[11] We can get a fuller view of the relation between release of narrative control and compassion by looking more closely at the way Pirandello develops the dramatic encounters that make up the substance of "A Character's Tragedy." Consider the grammatical forms in which these encounters are described. Italian is rich in idiomatic verbal constructions in which self is simultaneously subject and object. While not always so unequivocally reflexive in meaning as the paradigm "*Mi sono lavata la faccia*" ("I washed my face"), these idiomatic constructions place self in the grammatical relation of being simultaneously actor and acted-upon. The Italian in "A Character's Tragedy" abounds in these verb forms, as well as similar constructions rendering what English-speakers would think of as the subject of a sentence into the indirect object of an impersonal verb (thus: "it is pleasing to me" instead of "I like it"). While such locutions are generously present in Pirandello's prose overall, and are one of the factors that make him so hard to translate, in "A Character's Tragedy" they serve the special purpose of placing Pirandello the narrator on a par with the characters. He informs us at the outset that during his weekly audiences, "It happens to me [*m'accade*; impersonal verb with indirect-object pronoun] almost always to find myself [*di trovarmi*; infinitive with reflexive pronoun] in bad company."[12] Right from the beginning, Pirandello underscores his relative lack of control by employing the grammatical forms of a passive victim. Although they are his characters they are introduced to us as pushing rudely into his study. They are troublesome and outstay their welcome; he appears to be as much at their mercy as they at his.

The grammatical forms Pirandello employs in "A Character's Tragedy" reinforce situational elements that further undermine the distinction between an active narrator fully in control of the story and passive characters subject to the narrator's every whim. Consider, for example, the circumstance in which Pirandello places Dr. Fileno: as a character created by another author, he first appears on the scene with a presumed existence independent of and prior to Pirandello's dealings with him. Even more significantly, consider Pirandello's insertion of himself into the story as a character alongside his other characters. He is the narrator, all right, but he does not tell his story from the detached and distanced perspective of a Toti or Fileno. Instead, he enters, literally, into the tale as he tells it—in effect converting a narrative discourse into dramatic interaction even while still using a narrative form.

Pirandello made the move from narration to drama on several occasions in the course of his career, first writing a short story on a topic and then expanding it into a play. *It* Is *So! (If You Think So)* was originally the short story, "Mrs. Frola and Mr. Ponza, Her Son-In-Law." One of Pirandello's most famous plays, *Six Characters in Search of an Author*, is a dramatized development of themes first introduced in "A Character's Tragedy" and "Think it Over, Giacomino!" While in the case of "Think It Over, Giacomino!" the themes persist, the characters do not. Unlike Ponza and Frola, Dr. Fileno and Professor Toti never get beyond their inaugural stories. Neither one is the stuff of real dramatic participation. The characters in a drama become who they are through their interactions with others—other characters, the audience, the playwright who initially develops them, the director, actresses and actors who interpret them, and so on. Precious little room is allowed for the distanced independence and control to which Fileno and Toti aspire. Pirandello ends "A Character's Tragedy" by dismissing Fileno in favor of other characters who, whatever their faults, do not have Fileno's "wild ambition."[13]

And Pirandello himself? When Fileno first begins to suspect he is not going to be taken on as one of Pirandello's characters, he briefly considers the possibility that Pirandello may have scruples regarding the rights of the original author. Fileno dismisses these scruples as insignificant. For Pirandello, apparently, they are not insignificant; that other authors exist with their own stories to tell is something he thinks it significant to honor. This last point should be underscored, for it suggests a different and more humane form of distancing than we have discussed so far in this paper. In telling his story, Pirandello paradoxically places himself inside the story at the same time as he steps back to see himself from outside as just one storyteller among many. This self-aware form of distancing, which allows him to acknowledge what he is doing even as he does it, has a different feel about it than the more self-protective forms of distancing displayed by Toti and Fileno. Instead of cutting Pirandello off from affective entanglements with others, it plunges him into an affectively loaded encounter in which no one perspective manages neatly to subsume any other.

"A Character's Tragedy" echoes *It* Is *So! (If You Think So)* in its willingness to sacrifice narrative coherence to the affective possibilities inherent in dramatic interaction. It also provides a further gloss on Signora Ponza's claim to be, for herself, "nobody." Pirandello, in advertising himself as a compassionate storyteller, has more in common with Signora Ponza in this regard than might at first appear. Pirandello's compassion for his characters is born of a degree of narrative distance; no stories or plays would be written were this not the case. But he adopts a distance to put himself most effectively at his characters' disposal. In his dealings with the characters (not often "my" characters!), Pirandello says:

> I listen to them all with infinite forbearing; I take down each one's name and circumstances; I take into account their feelings and aspirations; I question them courteously and make the greatest possible effort to satisfy them; that is, to accept them in my own mind and in my writings just as they see themselves in their own mind as individuals.[14]

The attitude Pirandello describes here is startlingly reminiscent of Simone Weil's conception of a form of attention in which "the soul empties itself of all its contents in order to receive into itself the being that it is looking at, just as he is, in all of his truth."[15] The comparison suggests that seeing that the characters have their own stories to tell, stories different from the ones he might tell if left to his devices, frees Pirandello to attend so fully to others that, following Signora Ponza, he becomes for a time "nobody for himself."

Pirandello's brand of authorial attention, like Weil's metaphysical attitude, is at the least a precondition for compassionate response, if not itself a form of compassion. As a writer, the most effective expression of compassion he can offer the characters who visit him in his study is telling their stories in ways that make it possible for us, as audience, to feel for them even in cases where we find it difficult to feel with them. If his stories succeed in plunging us into the worlds of his characters so that we can accept them with compassion into our own minds, it will be largely because the devices Pirandello has employed as an author have communicated to us that he has already done as much himself. And, in the end, our responding in this way to his works will be the only proof Pirandello can give us that in portraying himself as a compassionate author he is not deluding either himself or us.

How the story is told is crucial. While the ability to step back and view himself from outside as one storyteller among many could have led Pirandello to adopt strategies protecting him from the challenges alternative perspectives might pose to his, the narrative devices employed in "A Character's Tragedy" seem to work in the opposite direction. Distancing, when self-aware instead of self-protective, paradoxically becomes the means to overcoming distance. However, when distancing fails to be self-aware its monstrous potentials are most likely to be realized. The historical narratives that Dr. Fileno constructs fail to reflect awareness that he is acting as narrator, and that the historical remotion allowing him to imagine the present as past is a narrative activity occurring in the present; to attend to this would make him susceptible again to the pain and suffering his philosophy of distance is designed to keep at bay. The epistemological remotion and crypto-solipsism inherent in much modern philosophy produces a philosophical narration similarly inattentive to the narration that is being constructed. In the act of articulating radical doubts about what others are thinking and feeling, or about what we are thinking or feeling ourselves, we presume much that we simultaneously claim to doubt. Yet our blindness to the contradiction is understandable. Attending too closely to these presumptions would so undermine the project of radical doubt that we would be left feeling more instead of less susceptible to error.

A form of distancing that reminds us of what we are doing as we construct a historical, philosophical, or other sort of narrative can reintroduce or even increase our vulnerability to those things—suffering or uncertainty, say—from which we sought protection through narrative distance. Yet, through the devices of style and situation he employs, Pirandello suggests that if we allow ourselves to acknowledge what we are doing as we do it, we can put narrative distance to more compassionate uses. This is not to say that it will always be necessary, or even possible, to go the lengths Pirandello went to in "A Character's Tragedy" to tell a story in a way that reflects an awareness of ourselves as narrators. Inserting ourselves into the stories we are telling as characters telling stories may in some cases be a cure worse than the disease, leading to a self-absorption that leaves us paralysed before the mirror. Interestingly, in *It* Is *So! (If You Think So)*, Laudisi's time before the mirror is neither emblematic of a permanent self-absorption nor an intermission in the action, but an episode that informs the way he interacts with the other characters in subsequent scenes. Nor should we forget that the Sunday morning interviews Pirandello describes in "A Character's Tragedy" are preliminaries to his writing the characters' stories—stories in which Pirandello by and large does not appear as a character himself.

If Pirandello's awareness of himself as one narrator among many enables him to transform the monstrous potentials inherent in narrative distancing into something more humane, his success has less to do with what he tells us about himself as author than the way he tells us things as an author—the stylistic devices he chooses and the way he sets scenes and introduces personages, doing everything possible to treat his characters as though they have lives of their own independent of his authorial control. His habit of transforming stories into plays is a further testimony to his willingness to let characters and stories develop outside the confines of his narrations, as he relinquishes his control over the dramatic realization to the autonomous decisions of directors and actors. And so, while Pirandello's clever trick of inserting himself into the text as a character alongside Dr. Fileno in "A Character's Tragedy" may lead us more explicitly to reflect on the differences between self-protective and self-aware distancing than the other devices he employs. Self-aware need not mean self-absorbed or self-conscious. Instead, at its best, self-aware distancing is the means by which we are able to begin looking beyond ourselves to cultivate a compassionate awareness of others.

3.

The message for us as persons, may be something like the following. One distinctive characteristic of persons is the ability to step outside the moment and view the world at some distance. On the face of it, "getting perspective on things" is a good idea, better than reacting in a series of unmediated instant responses. We devise useful explanations and interpretations, getting more and more adept, we hope, at the art of discovering—or constructing—meaning and value in our lives. Yet a sense exists in which the act of gaining perspective can be an act of mastery that extends beyond the immediate situation to other persons. "Yes, I can see your point of view," we might say. We would not usually add, "and therefore my point of view is more satisfactory, inasmuch as it subsumes yours." Yet that is often just what we assume—and when we do, our ability for distancing is fraught with all manner of monstrous potentials. While no simple formula exists for transforming the monstrous into the humane, if Pirandello has anything to teach us it may be that the transformation is unlikely to occur unless our distancing becomes self-aware in ways that work against pre-empting other perspectives. This means, in effect, placing our narrative voice alongside as opposed to above the voices of the other characters in the narration, transforming the narration into dramatic interaction in ways that make us vulnerable to suffering and uncertainty, but that also, if we are lucky, may over time make us truly human.

NOTES

1. Luigi Pirandello, "A Character's Tragedy," in *Eleven Short Stories/Undici Novelle: A Dual Language Book*, translated and edited by Stanley Appelbaum (New York: Dover Publications, 1994), p. 145.

2. *Ibid.*, p. 149.

3. *Ibid.*

4. Luigi Pirandello, *It* Is *So! (If You Think So)*, in *Naked Masks: Five Plays by Luigi Pirandello*, ed. Eric Bentley (New York: E.P. Dutton & Co., Inc., 1952), p. 66.

5. *Ibid.*, p. 68.

6. *Ibid.*, pp. 101-102.

7. Pirandello, “Think It Over, Giacomino!”, in *Eleven Short Stories*, p. 127.

8. Pirandello, *It* Is *So! (If You Think So)*, p. 129.

9. E. A. Robinson, “Eros Turannos,” (1916) in *Chief Modern Poets of England and America*, 4th ed., ed. G.W. Sanders *et al.* (New York: The Macmillan Co., 1957), pp. 46-47.

10. Pirandello, *It* Is *So! (If You Think So)*, p. 138.

11. Pirandello, “A Character’s Tragedy,” p. 147.

12. *Ibid.*, pp. 144-145.

13. *Ibid.*, p. 157.

14. *Ibid.*, p. 145.

15. Simone Weil, “Reflections on the Right Use of School Studies with an Eye to the Love of God,” in *Simone Weil Reader*, ed. George A. Panichas (Mt. Kisko, N.Y.: Moyer Bell, 1977), p. 51.

Seven

GOD, EVIL, AND THE MORAL SELF: THE AUGUSTINIAN ALTERNATIVE

Eric O. Springsted

When Hume critiques the rational weakness of religious belief on the problem of evil, he does so on the basis of a logical inconsistency he sees in theistic belief. Holding that God is both omnipotent and wholly good and admitting the obvious existence of evil in God's creation is not logically consistent, he maintains. While this problem has, since Hume and even before, continually exercised the wits of philosophers, it is not the only problem of evil. What might be called a religious problem of evil exists where the presence of evil threatens the moral resolve of believers, their ability to see goodness triumphing in the world and in their lives.

These two problems are not only two different sorts of problems. They also, I suggest, may ultimately bespeak two different conceptions of what the human will is for, and hence of the moral self. When the problem of evil is seen chiefly as a logical problem, the will is seen primarily as a power to choose; its best choice is informed by rational argument. That gives us a different sense of the moral self than in the other case, where a teleological cast exists to willing that is frustrated by evil and fulfilled only by the Good.

In this essay, I hope to show some of the differences just hinted at by examining Augustine's treatment of evil, primarily in his early *De Libero Arbitrio Voluntatis*.[1] I intend to show that while it is a philosophical defense of God's justice, it has another, perhaps more significant emphasis, a theological emphasis, in what Gilson calls "the search for God through the will."[2] Further, I argue that Augustine's view of the will, while controversial for contemporary thought, also provides a significant alternative to it with respect to our understanding of the moral self, to how we understand the problem of evil and finally to how faith itself might be understood.

1.

The issue at stake can be introduced by looking at Christopher Kirwan's recent treatment of free will in Augustine. Kirwan's book is a highly sophisticated discussion of Augustine's "free will defence," but which, at a crucial point, tends to assume Hume's point of view, and thus, I suggest, misses the overall goal of

Augustine's argument. But for that reason what is helpful is to see the distinctiveness in Augustine's argument.

In the course of examining Augustine's defence of free will Kirwan notes that the range of what Augustine must defend is obvious: human beings must be able to sin. However, he adds, the degree of that free will is problematic and, therefore, in the interest of saying something about how Augustine can defend God as a just punisher and a benevolent Creator, Kirwan distinguishes two germane degrees of freedom.[3]

The first is what he calls "freedom of spontaneity," or acquiescence. This degree of freedom allows that we have a will, that we own it and that it is not the result of compulsion. In the Stoic examples he gives, the will is the internal ability to accept our destiny as ours, even when the external result is the same, whether we acquiesce or not.

The second degree of freedom he notes is the freedom treated by Hume, when in the *Enquiry Concerning Human Understanding*, he defines freedom as: "By liberty, then, we can only mean a power of acting or not acting, according to the determinations of the will."[4] This sort of freedom, Kirwan explains, is a "two-way power"; that is, a single power to choose to do something or not to do something; "for which half of it the free man exercises depends on the determinations of his will."[5]

Kirwan is on firm ground by attributing both of the first two degrees of freedom to Augustine and in signalling their importance. The second is crucial to the case of defending God as a just punisher. Without freedom to defy the divine will and responsibility for bringing about states of affairs contrary to God's plan, difficulties exist in seeing how anyone can be justly punished.

However, if Kirwan is right in attributing both of the first two degrees of freedom to Augustine, I contend, and this brings us closer to our point, he has also glossed over two different kinds of freedom in discussing the two degrees. While a difference arises between degree number 1 where we can choose to acquiesce, and degree number 2 where we have a "double power" of choosing to act or of choosing not to act, that is not entirely the difference between the two freedoms. What we might call a hermeneutical difference between the two freedoms exists, for one has far more to do with what we might call "subjective intentions" and the other more to do with "objective intentions." What is at stake can be seen by looking at the classical sources Kirwan uses as illustration. For Hume does not add a degree of freedom that the Stoics miss; he has a different sense of the person and the will which causes him, and others who subscribe to the same sense of the self, to see the problem as they do.

The difference can be seen this way. For the Stoics, what is at stake in the freedom of the will is a question of our rationality, and because of this, our humanity. To acquiesce to fate—to will it for our own—is nothing more or less than choosing to accept our own providential role in the world as a whole. To choose our providential role and honor God by doing so is to be our true self. For example, Epictetus says: "If, indeed, I were a nightingale, I should be singing as a nightingale; if a swan, as a swan. But as it stands, I am a rational being, therefore I must be singing hymns of praise to God. This is my task; I do it, and will not desert this post, as long as it may be given me to fill it...."[6] This explains why Stoic conceptions of free will traditionally did not involve a double power; defiance made little sense. To will to defy the divine order with respect to our role may well be to cease having that role at all, and to play another, one belonging to a less than rational nature. It would be seen as becoming something else, which is why Epictetus warns: "Only consider at what price you sell your freedom of will."[7]

What is crucial for us to note is that here the issue of the will is fundamentally a moral one that is linked to what we are as persons. What is also significant is that discussions of the will in this context are far more concerned with a moral evaluation of what we might call the "inner person" than with any acts he or she may perform. That this is not so with a Humean conception of liberty is obvious from the context and content of Hume's own definition of liberty as the freedom to act or not act according to determinations of the will. Anyone who is at all familiar with the *Enquiry* knows Hume's intent. He is seeking to undo the Gordian knot of the metaphysical questions of the will and its causality all too quickly encountered in discussions of free will. He cuts the knot by pointing out that the question of freedom is not one of metaphysics, but a question of the ability to do or not do something. It has nothing to do with the metaphysical status of the will or with moral valuation. This is an impressive move. But at the same time we are impressed, we need to be aware that cutting the Gordian knot that way also does away with the picture of the person on which the Stoics relied. For Hume, or if not Hume then his followers, the person is, and only is, his or her public acts.

Kirwan is correct to suggest that Augustine has an operative conception of both degrees of freedom. But what is not apparent in Kirwan's discussion is that in which those degrees lie. For example, Kirwan establishes that the second degree of freedom is understood by Augustine through a discussion of power (*potestas*) in his works. But this still does not answer the question of "power for what?" A great deal depends upon how we answer this question, for it provides a clue to the nature of the will in Augustine and its purposes.

The question of "power for what?" asks whether we will take the power of the will to be most significantly an internal power, as the Stoics seemed to take it, or an external power, a power to act as Hume took it. The difference lies in whether we emphasize the power to accept or reject an argument or, more significantly, a world view, or the power to do or not to do something. This is a difference between conceiving the will as an internal activity that lies at the center of what a person is or conceiving it as the structure of uncoerced, publicly identifiable activity, which gives a different sense of the person.

Once we put it this way, though, we must recognize that the different kinds of freedoms are not mutually exclusive. They can be complementary, as long as we assume that a prior internal activity of willing somehow lays behind public activity. But if that is a picture that looms large in the popular mind, it also begs a question that many modern philosophers want to challenge. Following Hume's argument and an updated version of it given by Gilbert Ryle, it has been largely assumed that such an account involves a redundancy and an infinite regression, as it involves a (supposedly) quasi-causal account of the will to explain actions.[8] Ryle's argument suggests that to be consistent this account requires a cause for the will and a cause for that cause *ad infinitum.*

This argument is significant and will require a response later. But what we need to consider first is that, if Augustine sees the will as a matter of deciding between possibilities, the most significant choice is accepting or rejecting a designated view of the self and its relation to the world and God. What makes that choice crucial for Augustine is that this determines the moral quality of the will and person. It determines who we are. And that is a primary interest of his in the question of evil, for evil on this account is not just an unhappy state of affairs, but also a matter of assenting to that state of affairs. Or, better put, it is largely a matter of our subjective intentions within a state of affairs. This can be seen in the way Augustine talks about evil in *De Libero.*

2.

In the opening of *De Libero*, Evodius asks, "Is God the cause of evil?" This seemingly straightforward question is open ended in a way that Augustine exploits extensively. It poses a question about God's justice: "Evil exists in the world, that nobody denies; therefore, we ask, is God the cause of it?" A chief intent of *De Libero* is to answer this question by arguing that God is in no way to blame for evil, except the sort that one experiences in being punished justly. Although another way exists of taking this question and answering it. Ingenuously and non-rhetorically we can ask: "just where does evil come from?" That this sort of question was also in Augustine's mind is shown in his description of *De Libero* in the *Retractiones.* There he notes that this book was begun in Rome at a time when "we wanted to explore and discuss the origin of evil." In that discussion, he adds, "we concluded that the sole cause of evil lay in the free choice of the will," which was why he titled the book *On Free Choice of the Will.* I suggest, that while finding the origin of evil in the free choice of rational creatures exculpates God, a significant conclusion in itself, we miss Augustine's point in this treatise if we do not take seriously that the book also has another sort of conclusion, namely, a broader one about evil and the will. This other conclusion in turn affects how we understand the exculpation of God with respect to evil.

What this other sort of conclusion is and its importance can be seen by bearing in mind two things. The first is that Augustine did at an earlier time have another answer to the origin of evil that also vindicated God, that is Manichaeanism. The second is why he abandoned that answer. Augustine came to a newfound ability to think of God as immaterial, and, of equal significance, a realization that evil is not an external thing—an obstacle in our path—but a deformation, a privation of some good.

The point is this: if providing an argument that would exonerate God for bringing about a state of affairs were the whole problem, Manichaeanism is not a bad argument. Most people even have a psychological predisposition to it. The problem, though, as Augustine came to see it, is that evil is not as the Manicheans said. Evil is not an unfortunate state of affairs that can be recognized by just anybody; evil is not external to the thinker as the Manicheans assumed (that is somebody else's fault). It also has something to do with the person who sees that state of affairs as a problem.

This is then to say that Augustine has an entirely new way (for him) of thinking about where evil comes from, and that, in turn, forces him to think about what we call "the problem of evil" in a different light. This new light above all causes him to locate the site of evil within beings, that which is deformed, and it causes him to locate it at the point of their deficiencies. More existentially, what this must have forced Augustine to realize was that whatever else evil was, it was somehow a part of him, and that it was his deficiencies and not some external obstacle that constituted the problem. Nothing could be farther from Manichaeanism, ancient or modern, which, in effect, denies one's essential moral responsibility for who one is, and which blames it on external factors.

What is crucial to note here is that for Augustine the will, together with memory and intelligence, is something that is indispensably us. As Evodius says: "I find nothing which I can call my own if the will by which I accept or reject objects of choice is not my own will."[9] So, once he is in possession of a concept of the will and recognizes it as being integrally tied to who we are as persons, we may observe that no difficulty arises in stepping to the conclusion that moral evil has its root in the will.

But let us be careful to understand exactly how evil is rooted in the will. For it is two different, although not entirely unrelated things to say that the deficiency is in the act willed or to say the deficiency is in the willing will itself. And Augustine is worried about the willing will itself. As he says in discussing the evil of adultery: "Perhaps then lust (*libido*) is the evil element in adultery. As long as you look for evil in the overt act itself, which can be seen, you are in difficulty."[10] Similarly he argues that Adam's sin was something present in him even before he ate the apple.[11] What is also apparent is why Augustine is worried about the willing will itself for, not only does it color the external act, but, also, if evil is a privation of form, the will itself is deficient. Thus the problem of evil for Augustine is not only whether evil is logically compatible with God's existence, goodness, and creativity, but is also a problem of what we are.

To recognize that the will itself and its motions are what Augustine is most concerned about goes a long way toward explaining some features that many moderns find unsettling in reading *De Libero.* Chief among these is a lack of concern Augustine demonstrates towards the problem of suffering.[12] To be sure, he does not ignore it entirely. However, such a thorny problem as that of the suffering of innocent children is not even brought up until the closing chapters of the final book.[13] Even then the problem is only answered within the larger context of an argument that Augustine has been developing about the just order of the world. I do not think that Augustine was an insensitive man; indeed, far from it. Instead, the problem of suffering, of what happens to us, often unjustly, and which is, to us, the moral problem of evil is not the one with which Augustine is dealing. His problem is with the will itself.

But why this emphasis on the will itself? Whereas we moderns tend to take a "God's-eye view," a stance of complete objectivity toward knowledge, for Augustine one's moral knowledge is not something one has; it is, as assented to, what we are. So the questions of "whence evil?" and the compatibility of evil with God's goodness are also questions that involve self-knowledge. Reflection for Augustine is always morally reflexive. And as such questions of the moral order of the universe are also, at their root, questions of our own identity.[14] Therefore, Augustine is not only concerned with exculpating God in a work such as the *De Libero* but is also concerned, and perhaps most concerned to develop a sense of the moral person. His emphasis on what we are calling the internal motions of the will, instead of its outward powers, is crucial to his case. Or perhaps better put, God is exculpated precisely when we understand ourselves morally.

In Augustine's eyes the key issue becomes the direction of the will and that to which it assents. That is the problem of the moral self. And to the extent that this is his problem, this is not just a theoretical problem, but a spiritual one as well. Or, better put, all theoretical questions for Augustine are moral and spiritual questions. For the problem is not only one of explaining, say, to a neutral observer, how the will can be deficient in its willing and leaving it at that. This question also has existential interest for the inquirer. As such, the problem is that of redirecting the will of the inquirer through the course of argument so that it may will properly. Augustine claims: "In our journey of devotion, our goal is God. If therefore we think of him otherwise than as He is, our thinking compels us to walk in vanity, not blessedness...."[15] But not only is the goal that we should ultimately will properly, by so willing one should understand better also. The goal of right thinking is knowledge of God.

Thus I am claiming the deep purpose behind the *De Libero* is to get the soul to understand itself morally and to understand that it cannot understand itself morally unless it understands itself in relation to God. In this sense, Augustine's argument is a sort of *itinerarium mentis ad Deum*.

It is as such an *itinerarium* that we can make some general points about Augustine's argument as a whole. The argument, I suggest, may be less about God's morality in creating a universe where some evils occur and more a question directly posed to the will about its own moral stance towards the creation. As such the invitation is to disabuse our minds of what Leibniz was later to call our "anthropocentric conceit," the view that our desires are the basis on which the world order is formed. As Augustine himself put it in response to those who cavil about suffering: "They cannot see the highest good—what it is and how great it is—yet they wish everything to be the same as their idea of the highest good."[16]

The point I ultimately want to raise about Augustine's *De Libero* is this: the moral self is determined not so much by its public action or even potentiality for action as by the vision of the good to which it assents and to which it is thereby bound. Whether we assent to another as the center and orderer of the world or whether we make ourselves its moral center, that is what determines our moral self. But that further means that what is morally significant about us is our inner willing. The attempt to affect and purify that willing is the ultimate goal and cornerstone of Augustine's arguments in *De Libero.*

3.

If this is Augustine's position, difficulties exist for the modern philosopher in taking it seriously. First, as noted earlier, we have to contend with Hume's anti-metaphysical counter account of the will and Ryle's "ghost-in-the-machine" caricature of inner willing. Second, insofar as what is being willed and assented to for Augustine is an order of the universe, we are also led to ask whether all of Hume's objections in the *Dialogues concerning Natural Religion* about the fancifulness of most accounts of the order of the universe—that they lack proper epistemological justification—don't apply here.

Hume's and Ryle's arguments must be taken seriously. They also must be taken in context. The "ghost-in-the-machine" criticism is an apt caricature of a designated position that understands the will as an inner activity needed to explain outer activity or to characterize it as free or moral. But, as Stephen Clark has argued, accounts of inner activity are not always explanations for voluntary activity.[17] Moreover, as Iris Murdoch has suggested, while this argument is "perfectly sound over a certain range,"[18] it does not mean that an act of the will is not "an introspectible movement....(whose only structure) is its outer structure."[19]

So what is crucial to ask is whether Augustine's position is hopelessly metaphysical in the bad sense of the word, an unwarranted explanation for a perfectly normal phenomenon. I think not; on the contrary, it recognizes some crucial root concerns, especially moral ones, of human identity. What is "metaphysical"—and metaphysical elements are present in Augustine's thinking—in this case becomes something more like a matter of articulating this moral insight about human beings. A later generation has forgotten the original impetus for the thought that comes to see it as something other than what it was meant to be.

What, therefore, is Augustine's insight that needs to be preserved? First, his insight is that questions about the will are moral and spiritual questions, and that moral and spiritual questions insofar as they are linked to our sense of self are not always secondary to questions of so-called "objective" knowledge. In many instances these moral and spiritual questions often shape and configure questions of fact. The question of who we are is a moral question and bespeaks a fundamental moral struggle of the human being. As such we struggle with ourselves to know about the order of the world in which we live and struggle to put ourselves in some kind of larger order. The order we assent to is crucial to our self understanding, and hence to a best account of the moral person.

But here the modern philosopher may well ask: "Why not just worry about these consequences and evaluate them on their own merits, instead of on the basis of a private vision?" Or the philosopher may ask: "Why this vision and not another, if either can produce the same result?" Or even: "Is not this concern with the internal motions of the will an unholy fascination with one's self?" The answer to the last question is "No," precisely because our assent not only has consequences in act, but also produces the quality of our evaluations, and affects what we take to be valuable.

To assent to a moral vision is to evaluate life in a distinctive way, and to bind our will to a definite direction. In this way the internal motions of the will are not otiose, but are of primary importance to our standing as moral persons. For what is at stake ultimately in the assent of the will to a moral vision are such things as whether, for example, we see ourselves as self-sufficient or dependent upon another. If anything morally substantial exists to us, what we will to think of ourselves is crucial to that substance. This inwardness is not self-obsession as this is not a matter of being closed in on oneself. Instead, this inwardness is a sense of oneself in relation to others—a sense of openness.

The second of Augustine's insights I wish to highlight—and this responds to Hume's criticisms about the fancifulness of claims about the order of the world—is that this assent and the moral and spiritual struggle it implies are at the heart of what faith is. Conversely, faith is itself a fundamental human question for Augustine. Just what is at stake here can be seen by looking at Hume's characterizations of faith.

In the *Dialogues,* two conversants have faith: Demea, who gleefully believes a whole set of things about the universe without evidence, and Philo, who believes fewer things, but believes them on bad or weak evidence. In the essay on "Miracles" in the *Enquiry Concerning Human Understanding*, faith itself is ironically taken as the greatest example of a miracle because good epistemological sense dictates against the probability of what is believed. In both the *Dialogues* and the *Enquiry*, therefore, faith is taken as blind willing, blind assent to what reason shies away from affirming. Or, as Ambrose Bierce put it, "faith is belief without evidence in what is told by one who speaks without knowledge, of things without parallel."

Augustine understands that faith involves beliefs that cannot be proved. We also gain a sense that, at the time he wrote *De Libero*, he is seeking to assent to an order of the universe which we would now regard as highly fanciful. For at this time at Cassiciacum shortly after his conversion he began a project, of which *De Libero* was a part, of showing how all the liberal arts led to the knowledge of God. Therefore, he is subject to Hume's criticism of cosmologies. But that is not all that he is doing, nor even, at the deepest levels, what he is primarily doing. For he is not primarily seeking evidence for the order of the universe; he is ultimately trying to bring his identity into conformity with whatever that order is as being God's will. One of the key arguments in *De Libero* is the so-called ideological argument where Augustine moves from sense to inner sense to reason to show that his knowledge and being depends upon another who is greater than he. The heart of that argument is, I suggest, to bring his identity into conformity with the order of God and the soul uncovered by the argument. In it the particulars of the universe are not at question; only two items are involved, God and the soul. The question is how one relates oneself to that on which all else depends. That relation for Augustine is the real heart of faith; faith is not belief without evidence.

We must understand that as being at the heart of Augustine's project because that relation to God is what Augustine continues to ponder and struggle with for the rest of his life. The intellectualistic liberal arts project was soon given up; the struggle to conform with God's will was not. An impression arises that Augustine did not change many of his views on cosmology, nor given the expectations of his age should he have done so. But he did refocus the terms of that struggle with the will of God. Seven years after *De Libero* he wrote about assent in the *Confessions* in explicit terms of moral and spiritual struggle. The great commentary on John 4:15 presents in no uncertain terms the world perceived by the inner sense as the work of the eternal Word, and the self as having to listen and respond to that Word, especially as the Incarnate Christ. His great final work, *The City of God*, is a moral vision born of coming to understand himself and his world in the moral and spiritual terms of the Bible—and so the Bible itself in the terms of an historical human struggle with questions of who and whose we are.

Faith for him was not belief in what mind could not or did not know, as it appears to be for Hume and much of philosophy of religion after Hume. It was the moral and spiritual struggle of the will, in conjunction with the memory and intellect, to bring himself into conformity with God. Taken in conjunction with Augustine's first insight—that this moral struggle of the will is at the heart of our identity—we come to see what is at the heart of Augustine's philosophical enterprise. This is a different vision than the modern one. But this vision is also different from what is often characterized in modern philosophy, for this is not a case of bad metaphysics, but has an underlying moral seriousness—a sense that philosophy matters to how we will turn out—that much modern philosophy lacks. For the moral order to which we assent makes us who we are, and that, I also maintain, is a far more significant question about the freedom of the will than any other.

Something mysterious surrounds this inner quest, insofar as it is something to which public reason and method have no direct access. But it is not, for all that, incomprehensible or unheard of, as Augustine knew well. It may well be at the root of the common enterprise of understanding who we are. For as Augustine writes in the *Commentary on John*:

> Give me a lover, and he feels what I say. Give me one that longs, one that hungers, one that is travelling in this wilderness, and thirsting and panting after the fountain of his eternal home; give such, and he knows what I am talking about.[20]

NOTES

1. Augustine, *On Free Choice of the Will*, translated by A. Benjamin and L. H. Hackstaff (Indianapolis: Bobbs-Merrill, 1964).

2. Etienne Gilson, *The Christian Philosophy of St. Augustine* (New York: Random House, 1960), Part 2.

3. Christopher Kirwan, *Augustine* (London: Routledge, 1989), pp. 83-88.

4. David Hume, *Enquiry Concerning Human Understanding*, Book 8, Sc. 73.

5. Kirwan, *Augustine*, p. 85.

6. Arrian's *Discourses of Epictetus*, Bk. 1, ch. 16.

7. *Ibid.*, Bk.1, ch. 2.

8. G. Ryle, *The Concept of Mind* (London: Hutchinson, 1949), ch. 3, "The Will."

9. Augustine, *De Libero Arbitrio Voluntatis*, Book 3, ch. 1, v.12.

10. *Ibid.*, Book 1, ch. 3, v.20.

11. *Ibid.*, Book 3, ch. 24. See also Augustine, *De Genesis ad Litteram*, Bk. 11, ch. 5.

12. G. Bonner, *St. Augustine of Hippo: Life and Controversies* (1963, reissued Norwich: The Canterbury Press, 1986), p. 211.

13. Augustine, *De Libero Arbitrio Voluntatis*, Book 3, ch. 23.

14. Charles Taylor, *Sources of the Self: The Making of the Modern Identity* (Cambridge, Mass.: Harvard University Press, 1989), p. 137.

15. Augustine, *De Libero Arbitrio Voluntatis*, Book 3, ch. 21, v. 201.

16. *Ibid.*, Book 3, ch. 23, v. 233.

17. Stephen R.L. Clark, *A Parliament of Souls* (Oxford: Oxford University Press, 1990), p. 64.

18. Iris Murdoch, *The Sovereignty of Good* (New York: Schocken Books, 1971), p. 15.

19. *Ibid.*, p. 13.

20. Augustine, *In Joannis Evangelium Tractatus*, Book 26, ch.4.

Eight

THE POLITICS OF PERSONS: PASTORAL CARE AND THE CHRISTIAN TRADITION

Tony Dancer

When I speak of the "politics of persons," I do not do so in the contemporary and popularized sense, which restricts its meaning to "professional" or parliamentary politics. Instead, such politics have to do far more with what Jens Glebe-Möller has described as "discussions and decisions concerning how societies and individuals should organize their life," applicable to all of humanity, in all our "amateurness."[1] Politics, therefore, have to do with the form of life in which a person moves, establishes, contributes, and takes part. My thesis is that pastoral care in the Christian tradition is one primary way in which politics such as Glebe-Möller describes are manifested, made known, and taught. The politics of being a person are made known most fully in the process and content of pastoral care, and therefore are central to the identity of what it means to be human, and, in this instance, Christian.

Pastoral care's political importance arises because good pastoral care is affective care, being pedagogical and thus formative in both its shape and structure. However, Christian pastoral care has forsaken its own tradition and adopted that of modernity, namely, its psychotherapeutic and philosophical understanding of being a person. However, the affective nature of care and the tradition in which it belongs are, I believe, enmeshed. I wish to suggest that a more apt and appropriate approach is for Christianity to recover its own distinctive tradition or identity of pastoral care, but to do so not with an ear to modernity. Only then will it be able to provide appropriate, affective care again; care that has both a focused vision and understanding of its own form of life, and is able to engage persons and the world accordingly.

This chapter seeks to outline the gulf that separates pastoral health care from the Christian tradition, and to explore ways to think across it. To this end, the chapter is an introduction to a problem in Christian pastoral care that has some bearing on the discussion of how we understand what it is to be human, and what makes for appropriate care. My underlying assertion is that Christian pastoral care has its own Christologically determined identity that embodies in its practice an understanding of the reality of personhood, and that this has something positive and significant to offer for us. The sort of care I speak of recovers "difference" as a necessary feature of personhood and pastoral care, and proposes that this distinction is not only helpful but liberating, providing the basis for the freedom to become.

1. World-Views and Being Human

Pastoral care is of central practical importance to the Christian faith, being the way most people will experience both faith and the Church, and as such is one of faith's primary self-expressive acts. Its form and content, and most distinctively its understanding of being human, were recast under the influence of the Enlightenment, and this paradigmatic lynch-pin of what is understood as being a person, I will now explore.

At the heart of pastoral care is the question: what does it mean to be human? Being human is about being a person, and being a person is not a presence of mind, or an idea, but a concrete, experiential, and pedagogical reality. The person is the place in which our past history and our future hopes collide and are reconciled in the social matrix of our lives. Those familiar with it may see similarities of this view with the learning cycle, which expresses the process of learning as a cyclical movement from practice, through exploration, reflection and response, back to practice. Such a cycle is engaged and encountered by effective pastoral care.

The parameters for our understanding of what it means to be human, or a person, are largely determined by our world-view. In turn, the understanding of being human which the carer holds to be true and applicable, directly affects the content and shape of the pastoral care which is delivered. In other words, our vision of the fullness of humanity is both behind and before us as we engage and shape another's life, being paradigmatic for care. Our understanding of persons is directly affected by our "primary narrative"—the abiding story or world-view that makes sense of reality as normative and coherent for our existence. Consequently, our understanding of persons is informed directly by one, and perhaps indirectly by many, primary narratives. Where more than one narrative informs our understanding, some formal hermeneutical or interpretive decision must be made with regards to organizational priority of one primary narrative, or perspective, or world-view, above others.

However, the limitations of a particular world-view does not necessitate relativism, for that would be to deny the belief in the universal significance and truth of the position we hold. Instead, such limitations try to acknowledge the limits of being human when it comes to knowing the truth. It revolves around the priority of praxis for knowledge, such that knowing comes primarily not from thinking, but from doing or acting; the "real" takes precedence over the "ideal." Acting then, is the basis of being, and such actions are culturally bound—be it religious culture (for example, Church and its doctrine) or the wider culture (for example, state laws, social codes of conduct, linguistic cultures, and information technology). The reality of world-views and their influence on personhood is what forms the backdrop for the problem of Christian pastoral care.

2. Pastoral Care and Modernity

Modernity and Christianity have never been the easiest of partners. In its desire to reject and overcome the restricting presence of Christendom, modernity relocated reality and provided a new primary narrative or world-view for navigating around it. In order to understand the problem in relation to pastoral care, we must look briefly at one facet of the Enlightenment: the turn to the subject and the knowledge of the self.[2]

The Enlightenment replaced the universal unifying world-view of faith with what were thought to be "objective," "enlightened-apprehensions" of humanity as the universal and unifying perspective upon reality. With it, reality became that which could be empirically verified or scientifically proved, and human autonomy became the ideal form of perceiving and controlling reality. The mind of the individual, embellished in reason, became the final arbiter of reality, and with it philosophy reigned supreme. Reason was acclaimed as the universal perspective upon reality mediated not by faith, but by the autonomous individual through verifiable apprehensions of rationality. The self became the final arbiter of reality, and human autonomy the prize. Two distinct realities emerged; one of faith, one of reason, with faith being predominantly made subservient to reason.[3]

Through the emphasis on autonomy, the axis for our knowledge of God, and so our knowledge of being human and of reality, shifted from the vertical to the horizontal; from revelation to reason. Religious communities became little more than a touch of tastefully added transcendence to the reality of reason. Significantly, being human, which was the axis upon which the Enlightenment turned, was redefined on rational autonomous grounds; an anthropological basis for God and reality which has continued to the present day.

This anthropological basis of knowledge was an appeal to the abstract qualities of the common reality of being human, and as Lowe has pointed out, it betrayed a perception of difference as opposition or competition instead of as distinction. It sought to overcome the dualist threat that difference was thought to pose by unifying reality and knowledge-of-reality around what was thought to be a common reality or theme: reality was unified around the rational being. It was thought that overcoming the opposition of difference in this way would provide the basis for peace and freedom. However, the opposite proved to be true. The result was a homogenous indifference that was perceived as unity, with the tragic consequence that our autonomy, our individuality, our variety and human freedom to be and become persons, was lost in this general, and often bloody so-called "unity." Genuine difference, and with it genuine freedom, was a casualty of the modernist paradigm, for the fuel of modernity is the dynamic of freedom-from, instead of freedom-toward. With the loss of difference our personal distinctiveness, our human particularity and individuality became irrelevant to who and what we are as persons. In modernity, humanity lost the ability to relate to the other, to those different from ourselves, and perceived such difference not as enriching, but as a direct threat to a person's unity, ideal, and identity. The mind, or the self, became the locus of reality's definition, perception, and control.

This situation brings itself to bear on Christian pastoral care most fully in the twentieth century, in which psychoanalysis was born and became the accepted practical science of the self. In the same way that theology has often sought to underpin itself with philosophy, pastoral care sought to retain its credibility and usefulness by rapturously adopting a psychoanalytic and psychotherapeutic method, practice, and understanding of the nature of being human—of being a person. Thereafter, at times little has existed to distinguish psychotherapy, counseling and Christian pastoral care. However, my suggestion is that this acceptance not only undermines the identity and effectiveness of Christian pastoral care, but undermines also the wider Christian identity and does not adequately provide for a positive account of being human, in all its diversity. By adopting such methods as the primary means of providing care, we undermine the foundations of freedom and fulfilment we wish to nurture, enable, and encourage.

Christianity is not without its own tradition of pastoral care; however, this was shed in the name of modernity. In the same way that faith in God has been subsumed under the wider cultural reality, so too theology and the Christian tradition have been squeezed out of the arena of the self. However, the identity of Christian pastoral care has its own tradition and identity. It has something significant to say and offers us a perspective upon being human, on being persons that are at once transcendent and immanent, at once other and with us, at once engaged in unity and difference.

3. Recovering Pastoral Care

In the light of modernity's dominance, some thinkers have called for the recovery of tradition; a recovery of a world-view and perspective internal to the Christian faith, both generated by and generative of it. These people seek to recover the distinct difference between Christian pastoral care and secular care—to recover a form of care that is derived from the world-view in which it is set. In this way, such approaches seek to reconcile modernity with the tradition, overcoming modernity's dominance and its inappropriate understandings of personhood and ways of dealing with difference.

Don Browning offers one of the most distinctive and well known attempts to recover this identity, in his attempt to recover what he calls the moral context of pastoral care.[4] His endeavors are governed by his desire that theology should be public and critical, and so take modernity seriously; his "moral context" is derived primarily from the arena of moral philosophy. Consequently, he overcomes the pastoral care's dependence on psychotherapy with a dependence on a philosophical meta-ethic in his attempt to mediate between modernity and faith. For Browning, personhood is philosophically and morally defined: being is primarily about doing, and the appropriate shape of doing is philosophically determined. However, he asserts that personhood is more than enacted morality, and includes, for example, spiritual and physical dimensions. In seeking to subsume these aspects under his general moral normative or unifying framework for the sake of unity or normativity, Browning fails to acknowledge the distinct diversity that is entailed in being human, and continues the modernist slide into homogeneous humanity. While to focus upon doing may be a helpful basis for pastoral care (breaking free, as it does, from the ideal of the mind), that our doing be philosophically determined is not appropriate. Tradition or identity is not recovered, but only relocated within Browning's moral philosophical perspective

A differing approach that acknowledges modernity, however, can be seen in what Martin Cook has called the "open confessional" approach.[5] This approach does not abandon the critical eye, but uses it in its Christian context, from where it can draw on other resources and address cultural issues. The approach is governed by submission to faithfulness, and a critical, realistic approach to the idealism of modernity. It overcomes the fear of the Other (as unknowable) by being open, without homogenizing the coherence of its own self-identity.[6] Consequently it can function on an *ad hoc* basis, as the spirit moves, instead of having the need for normative systematic speculation.

The key to pastoral care's identity lies in this coherence through inferential, descriptive methods, instead of the speculative deduction of Browning's experiential approach; within this approach, the integrity of difference and self-identity are maintained. Such an approach does not cease being public, but requires us to re-invest the notion of public faith with new meaning. Instead of an appeal to the public as "warrants available to any intelligent, reasonable, responsible person" we can and should conceive of it as understanding "a religion as fundamentally a public, communal activity, not a matter of the individual's experience."[7] With this change of emphasis, "publicness" can be seen as a social thing, and a thing which necessarily entails difference. The combination of being open and confessional makes it more apt and more fitting, especially in relation to pastoral care.[8] Only by being confessional, but also open (to ourselves and the "other"), can we acknowledge most fully the parochial nature of our knowing.

4. Proposals for the Political Person

In some concluding remarks, I would like to give some indication of what Christian pastoral care might look like, and consequently what it has to offer for enabling people to be persons, political persons, if it were to take seriously its own tradition, language of faith, public setting, and Christological basis. In other words, this is what Christian pastoral care might look like if it were to take seriously its own identity (world-view) as it engages others.

The Christian faith is a necessarily confessional tradition, locating pastoral care's identity (past, present, and future) within the context of private confession and public witness. As such it does not seek static practice of care, but a creative, *ad hoc* approach which is expressive of the spontaneity and diversity of the presence of Christ's spirit in the world, which the carer embodies. Living the life of the pastoral carer entails living life in Christ, by freedom, for freedom. Such a life enables difference and diversity to exist in harmony within the unity of our identity. The carer becomes the sign of and hope for what it is to be human, for the carer embodies the world-view, the text, the story, the presence of the Spirit in his or her presence with the person being cared for.

The shape this takes in practice is necessarily fluid, *ad hoc* and adaptable, diverse, and diffuse. However, if Christian self-identity is to take difference and diversity seriously in its own self-description, it has to be open to other interpretations of this tradition, and potential changes in practice and self-understanding this may bring, providing they do not undermine the foundations of faith. Adopting an understanding of "thick description," such as Clifford Geertz proposes, we might say that only through "thickening" our understanding of our tradition (our primary perspective of faith) with other perspectives, insights and people (being open to the other, be it discipline or person) can we become gradually more fully a person, and grow in the fullness of Christ.

Care is not primarily about moral action, nor about preaching the Word, but embodying the Spirit (who is with us) and witnessing to its reality in love for the neighbor; comforting, praising, rejoicing, celebrating, encouraging, and being in solidarity with the victim, that is, the person for whom we care. This is the life of living the promise; the life of embodying the memory. This is the life of care, giving space for the "other" to develop, by relating to, rebuking, confronting, sharing with, and most of all listening to the other. In the witness which is care, we embody through grace the reality of life in Christ, and so hold together the diversity of care and its contexts, enabling people and society to respond and be transformed—becoming more fully human and more fully free.

Furthermore, such care is open. This openness looks forward to a pastoral care which calls us to take a broken and war-torn world seriously, but to do so with joyful vision; to face its reality but look beyond its tragedy. Pastoral care, in all its thickness, calls for a joyful, hopeful, faithful vision grounded in a realist vision of faith that is empowered by and empowering through the spirit. Such care is generative of a humanity, a notion of personhood, which is grounded in the same vision. Such care demands a theology which is "lively, ecstatic theology, that dances, puzzles, stimulates, delights, strikes sparks from contemporary experience and transforms individuals and communities...filled with a sense of power, promise, and expectation."[9]

Power, promise, and expectation are at the heart of the Christian faith, seen paradigmatically in the death/resurrection sequence. The reality of this power, promise and expectation is lived, by faith, in the practice of the carer. The comic practice of openness provides hope. While the comic may look out of place in a world which is forever taking itself seriously, I believe it resides at the heart of care, and of our humanity. The comic is the basis of hope, for laughter has the power to erode injustice. It enables us to see the comic nature of the seriousness with which we confront the world—for the world is not the end of the matter; laughter is hope's last weapon in the face of the world—the place where God is most God and most immanent, and we are most aware of the fact, and most human. The irony of seriousness gives rise to the comic encounter.

We must recover the comic vision of our redemption in Christ, the irony of God doing the humanly impossible in human form, the futility of our own attempts to achieve the same, and Christ's refusal to become a cosmic projection of our own values, embodying the comic declaration that God has reclaimed us as his. This is the joke we embody in our care, a care which can do no better than to recover the humor of eschatological grace through the freedom of the spirit, such that people may be more free to be themselves—and laugh.

In summary: I am proposing that pastoral care's identity is to be found most fully in diversity (of which comedy is an example). The unity of identity which care seeks is expressed or embodied most fully and most appropriately in Christ, and so in us in-Christ, and not in the tenants of modernism. Being human is most appropriately Christologically, instead of anthropologically determined, and pastoral care can provide the Christian tradition with perhaps the most adequate means of actualizing such humanity.

I suggest that if Christ is truth, present with us as the basis for and content of our care then we must move away from modernist desire to recast notions of humanity and recover our diverse, creative, and fluid notion of our experience of Christ that quickens and empowers our being. However, it does so in a way which is open, taking seriously diversity as difference, not opposition. Relating to difference in this way is itself liberating, and again enables pastoral care and the Christian life to reach out and engage other people(s) appropriately and publicly in love and to leave behind our heritage of clerically or even ecclesially bound understandings of care as witness which betray not only a misunderstanding and consequent fear of difference, but also a static and parochial misunderstanding of salvation. This is a care which is publicly and privately engaged, both individually and socially transformative. My hope is that revisioning care in this way may begin to restore the joyful presence of the re-creative God at the heart of pastoral care's method and practice, and at the heart of being human.

NOTES

1. Jens Glebe-Mölle, *A Political Dogmatic* (Philadelphia: Fortress, 1987), p. 9.

2. Walter Lowe, *Theology and Difference: The Wound of Reason* (Indianapolis: Indiana University Press, 1993).

3. Ingolf Dalferth, *Theology and Philosophy* (Oxford: Blackwell, 1988).

4. Don S. Browning, *A Fundamental Practical Theology* (Minneapolis: Fortress, 1991); (ed.) *Practical Theology* (Minneapolis: Fortress, 1983); *The Moral Context of Pastoral Care* (Philadelphia: Fortress, 1976).

5. Martin Cook, *The Open Circle: Confessional Method in Theology* (Minneapolis: Fortress, 1991).

6. See also John Thiel, *Nonfoundationalism* (Minneapolis: Fortress, 1994), pp. 92-94.

7. William Placher, "Revisionists and Postliberal Theologies and the Public Character of Theology," *The Thomist*, 49 (July 1985), pp. 392-416 (p. 407).

8. See Bruce Marshall, "Absorbing the World: Christianity and the Universe of Truths" in *Theology and Dialogue*, ed. Bruce Marshall (Notre Dame, Ind.: Notre Dame University Press, 1990), pp. 69-104.

9. Stephen Pattison and James Woodward, A *Vision of Pastoral Theology: In Search of Words that Resurrect the Dead* (Edinburgh: Contact Pastoral, 1994), pp. 3-4.

Nine

HIV AND RELIGION: TOWARD A NEW DIALOGUE

Margaret J. Morris

Public Health Medicine's pragmatic responses to preventing transmission of the human immunodeficiency virus (HIV) are premised on principles of universal access to information, treatment, and care.

Access can be thwarted not only by inadequate resources but also by personal and corporate philosophies and traditions which authorize and disguise discriminatory practices. When the proscriptions, for example, placed by religions on gay identities and lifestyles, on the freedom and status of women, and on the entitlement of young people to sexual health information are considered in the context of HIV prevention, universal access to information, treatment, and care is vulnerable.

A serious public health issue drives an engagement with social and religious taboos and in so doing exposes the potential for conflict between the principles of mutual respect for diverse identities which underpin philosophies of universal access and the need to protect the health communities. This chapter identifies and explores the place of religion in some often hidden institutional aspects of the conflict.

1. The Virus

During 1981, clusters of a rare pneumonia, *pneumocystis carinii* and a cancer, Kaposi's Sarcoma, were reported in the USA. A steadily increasing number of cases, the earliest all involving young gay men, attracted the attention of the medical and scientific worlds and were ultimately recognized as the first identified instances of what became known as Acquired Immune Deficiency Syndrome or AIDS.

AIDS is a syndrome which occurs in the wake of the immunity-suppressing activity of a virus, HIV. This hypothesis is challenged by some, but experienced researchers are in virtually unanimous agreement, underscored during 1995 by the results of a British study. For the purposes of this chapter the orthodox view is accepted.[1]

The human immunodeficiency virus is a retrovirus, which, like other viruses, can replicate by incorporating into a host cell its own genetic material, its DNA or Deoxyribonucleic Acid. However, the life cycle of a retrovirus includes an additional stage because the genetic material is stored in a molecule known as RNA (Ribonucleic Acid) and not in DNA. The retrovirus is required to convert its RNA to DNA, making the virus more difficult to detect but providing the process with an identifiable and distinct point of intervention, the enzyme reverse transcriptase, which researchers seek to exploit in the development of treatments through both virological and immunological sciences.

The receptor cells to which HIV binds and eventually destroys or infects are found on, among others, those cells which play a key role in activating and co-ordinating a person's immune responses. HIV reduces the immune system's ability to protect a person from the impact of infections, both minor and serious. In the absence of other causes of immunodeficiency not attributable to HIV an AIDS diagnosis is occasioned by the presence of one or more opportunistic infections or tumors as defined by the Centers for Disease Control and Prevention. The definitions are appropriated and, in some instances, adapted by health agencies around the world, though environmental differences may reduce the usefulness of the definitions in some settings.[2] Not only does HIV replicate but it also confounds research programs and treatment regimes by its extensive variability; a variability of mutation and disease progression unique to each virus and to each individual experience of HIV infection.[3]

Transmission of the virus can occur when an exchange of HIV-infected body fluids takes place. The fluids are blood, semen, vaginal and cervical secretions, and breast milk. Although present in the tears and saliva of people with HIV, no transmission of the virus by these routes has been reported. Transmission occurs most commonly through unprotected penetrative anal or vaginal sex with a person who has HIV; by sharing injecting equipment with a person who has HIV; from a mother with HIV to her child either before or during birth or through breast feeding; and through the use of unscreened and untested blood, blood products, and transplant organs. A person with HIV can remain well for many years but may pass the virus to another person at any time after becoming infected if steps are not taken to prevent transmission.

Where it occurs, HIV, unlike other pandemics, affects the most economically and socially productive women and men: young adults and the middle-aged—the people to whom demographic units, socially cohesive networks, and institutional infrastructures on the micro and the macro scales look for stability and survival.

The extent of HIV's demographic and economic impact on some African communities has far-reaching implications for the global distribution of resources, especially those assigned for health care, education, trade, and industry. Africa has only 9 percent of the world's adults but has 67.7 percent of the world's adults with AIDS. Similarly disproportionate figures can be drawn from Latin America and the Caribbean.[4] More recent reports from Asia suggest that before long India will have replaced Africa as the pandemic's epicenter.[5]

Although great strides have been made in understanding the virus and developing treatment and care strategies, these are costly and not universally available. It remains the case that no cure or vaccine exists nor will one likely exist in the foreseeable future. Our generation has had to assume that HIV is here to stay.[6]

2. Religion Responding to HIV

In the face of such a global public health crisis imaginative, creative, and diverse responses are required which can: (1) develop and assign resources for more extensive and effective prevention and care programs; (2) include and draw on the experience of people directly affected by HIV; (3) take full account of prevailing epidemiological evidence and cultural traditions and identities. A maximization of responses is needed which requires the mobilization of all the resources which societies and communities can muster, including those of religion.

Institutional engagement with the global experience of HIV and AIDS may have far-reaching and difficult-to-discern implications. HIV is now well known for the relentless efficiency with which it destroys an individual's physical immune defenses, and is increasingly accredited with an ability to expose the weaknesses and strengths of societies' social, political, economic, and religious infrastructures. The ensuing tensions create a dilemma for religions responding to HIV and people affected by HIV. Should the virus be regarded as a health issue or a moral issue?

Set in an American context, Charles Perrow and Mauro F. Guillen's book *The AIDS Disaster* offers a comprehensive account of an array of competing social and moral forces which bear on any responses to HIV and AIDS. Their chapter on "Organisational Responses to AIDS" sheds light on the "condoms: reducing transmission versus encouraging promiscuity," and "the free needles: reducing infection versus encouraging drug dependency" type of debates which have immediate application into United Kingdom and global contexts.[7] The responses of religions and an understanding of the role they play in a global experience of HIV will rely on the institution's as well as the individual's discernment of realities.

Perrow and Guillen take the view that transmission of the human immunodeficiency virus can only be slowed and its effects minimized by strategies which take seriously the issues of social justice. These will include redressing inequities in access to health care, employment, housing, education and information, extending economic cooperation and fair distribution of financial, material and ecological resources and combating discrimination on the grounds of color, race, religion, gender, sexual orientation, physical or mental disability, and age.

In developing countries, for example, limited resources for basic health care result in low standards of hygiene and health education; both blood used for transfusions and blood products remain unscreened and untreated; needles for injecting are used on several patients before being discarded; access to clinical abortion, to contraception and to prophylactic condom supplies may be inadequate or unavailable. All are implicated in the exposure of individuals to the transmission of HIV, as is the relationship between the impact of the virus on women and on the status of women.

What is now recognized is that the health of communities depends largely on the health of women:

> Women's lack of status within the family and society heightens their vulnerability to infection (HIV) and other consequences of the pandemic. The stigma attached to AIDS can subject women to discrimination and other violations of their rights.[8]

For economic, cultural, and religious reasons, women may have little or no control over their own health. Different standards of sexual behavior for men and women and the pressure to conceive and bear children may accelerate the spread of the virus:

> In unprotected intercourse women have a greater chance than men of being infected with HIV... AIDS campaigns should join forces with campaigns to raise women's social and economic status.[9]

Yet such campaigns will meet resistance from both women and men where respectable status and identity are defined by traditional practice. For example, in societies where clitoridectomy is practiced, unexcised women are not regarded as "real" women and are marginalized. Consequently, women can be placed under intense pressure to conform. "How could I not do it since I live here?"[10] Where initiation is a central dimension of the practice or where a family's or husband's honor is at stake, levels of resistance to change may be high and both culturally and religiously inappropriate.

In her book, *AIDS and its Metaphors*, Susan Sontag brings other tensions and issues into sharper focus. Sontag illuminates obfuscation and diversity and succeeds in demonstrating that responses to HIV and AIDS, instead of being uniform and homogeneous, cannot be separated from diverse and differing contexts; diversities and variabilities which themselves generate the tensions and obfuscation to which metaphors point, and, if successfully de-coded, expose. Her insight discloses, for example: (1) the difficulties of getting noticed that which and those whom individuals and societies prefer to ignore; (2) the well-being of people affected by HIV can be assured neither by visibility nor by invisibility, but may be by either or both; (3) the design of strategic responses to HIV is required to take account of multiple interconnected histories, memories, and realities.[11] Reflecting on the shame and guilt often felt by a person with HIV, Sontag illustrates these dichotomies and captures the complexities by writing:

> the illness flushes out an identity that might have remained hidden from neighbors, job-mates, family, and friends. It also confirms an identity and, among the risk group in the United States most severely affected in the beginning, homosexual men, has been creator of community as well as an experience that isolates the ill and exposes them to harassment and persecution.[12]

Similar bifurcation can be discerned in Thom Gunn's poem "Sacred Heart".[13] Gunn's images from a street in San Francisco are no less relevant than the gospel images from that road to Jericho (Luke 10:29-37). They are reflected again in the calls of religions for generous, self-giving, non-judgmental responses on the part of individuals, communities, and entire societies in the face of HIV and AIDS and in calls for chastity, fidelity, monogamy, and celibacy. The one offers an opportunity to claim HIV as a universal concern, as "our" concern; the other a means to scapegoat and blame and as justification for avoidance and denial: this is not "my" concern or the concern of "my" people, but "their" concern and their own fault. This reflects a tension noted by the Archbishop of Canterbury, Dr. George Carey, speaking at the Department of Health and Oxford Regional Health Authority's jointly sponsored conference of 1994 "HIV/AIDS/Sexual Health and Britain's Faith Communities." He posited that "honesty causes the Christian Churches and other faith communities to ask whether we are part of the answer or part of the problem."[14]

Calling for more of the compassion and humility he believes to be present in most faith communities the Archbishop refers to the "ironic combination of amoral and hedonistic cultural norms with streams of puritanical moralism, engendering furtiveness, and moral suspicion."[15]

If responding to HIV solely as a health issue is impossible, HIV will rarely be experienced solely as a health matter. Uncovering and understanding the HIV experience is an appropriate task for religious groups, but in the UK most of us have yet to meet someone living with HIV; most of us have not known someone who has died with AIDS. The invisibility of people affected by HIV can reinforce notions that HIV need not concern us or our community, our congregation or our Church.

But many hundreds involved in social services, health services, education and in voluntary agencies, in city and county policy-setting and decision-making processes as well as people with HIV infection and those closest to them, are confronting issues around HIV on a regular basis. By and large, faith groups choose not to involve themselves, with the result that people affected by and living with HIV still hear religion offering only judgmental and ill-informed responses to questions asked and issues raised. Sontag might ask whether the comfort-inducing convenience of a perception that equates invisibility to absence can or should be reversed.

Faith groups of some sort have a presence in most communities, often with access to national and international organizational resources and networks. Can they, or should they be persuaded that they have a major contribution to make in raising awareness and in creating a climate in which transmission of the virus can be slowed and in which people affected by HIV and AIDS can access support without fear of stigmatization and isolation? Encounters with HIV and AIDS raise questions at personal and at societal levels, questions which require a comprehensive and informed engagement if religion (any religion, but here I refer especially to Christianity) is to address adequately the diverse tensions and dichotomies which HIV exposes.

But for us to engage comprehensively and informedly people affected by HIV, including those with a Christian faith, we will have to be able to make their experiences and their reflections on them known and available to the Church. But is the Church prepared to accept their gifts of theological, pastoral, and liturgical challenge? Or, to use a different language, how can the Church recognize that the Church has AIDS? That the body of Christ has AIDS?

To many the image of Christ's body with AIDS will be anathema, but traditional and relevant Christian "body" language facilitates the appropriation of a counseling model to address dialogically and more adequately some of the difficulties and tensions which HIV exposes and which at the same time can make known an experience of HIV. References to counseling assume a psycho-dynamic model.

3. Counseling Church

Before it can ascertain the realities and acknowledge the tensions, a Church with HIV must listen both to itself and also to a world with HIV. It must engage a new dialogue and be prepared for a complex interplay of values and emotions compounded by moral, ethical, and theological contradictions. It must ask, who is the Church on the road to Jericho? The abandoned and bruised one? The outcast helper? Or the passerby?

Before the Church can ascertain the realities and acknowledge the tensions it needs "ears" which can enable the institution to listen to its own "base-line—what is not openly said, but possibly being felt";[16] "ears" which can also be the Church as counselor for persons affected by HIV.

In his book, *Still Small Voice,* Michael Jacobs devotes an entire chapter to the principle that psycho-dynamic counseling is informed by the wisdom of understanding through self-knowledge. He is concerned that such wisdom should characterize all good counseling training and practice. He writes:

> Counselors need the skills but skills alone are not sufficient. They also need to be aware of the conscious and hidden factors in themselves which influence others. It is therefore essential that we prepare ourselves for this work by beginning a continuous self-examination which underpins all the technical learning. Since the pastor sees self-knowledge as one of the aims of his counseling the client, he cannot expect less of himself. 'Physician, heal thyself.'[17]

For the relationship between a Church-with-HIV's self-understanding and the counsel and care it offers to people affected by HIV to be mutually beneficial, the Church is called to listen attentively to the feelings of its institutional self/selves (for the corporate must take account of the individual) and to the experiences and feelings of the world it inhabits, a world affected by HIV.

Applying the following quotation from the World Health Organization's (WHO) *Guidelines for Counseling about HIV Infection and Disease* to the Church as institution and as organization as well as to an individual, helps us to imagine the impact HIV will have on the Church during the coming years:

> A diagnosis of HIV infection or AIDS, or a suspicion or recognition of the possibility of infection, brings with it profound emotional, social, behavioural, and medical consequences.... Adjustment to HIV infection involves constant stress management and adaptation. It is a dynamic, evolutionary, and lifelong process that makes new and changing demands on the infected individuals, their families, and the communities in which they live.[18]

Listening to and reflecting upon these stressful environments and experiences can inform and be informed by the psycho-dynamic tools of analysis and appraisal. An application of psychoanalyst Wilfred R. Bion's ideas allows an exposure of the tensions, focused primarily in the pastoral/authoritarian dichotomy, facing organizations, institutions, and individuals in the management of HIV-related stress and change.

4. Counseling a Changing Church

In his post-World-War II psychoanalytical studies of groups, Bion noticed the intense emotional activity which influences a group's behavior. He recorded how the completion of a group's task is often obstructed, even thwarted, by emotions of anxiety, fear, love, and hate. He named the sources for these emotions "basic assumptions,"unconscious responses to early life relationships which he divided into three categories: dependency, fight/flight, and pairing.[19] Bion argued that these unconscious assumptions underlie all group behavior; and he demonstrated how they influence a group's choice of leadership, its orientation to events, and its capability to deal effectively with the task to which it ostensibly is addressed.

Change, especially major change, and its attendant sense of loss, awakens intense emotional responses which may threaten, according to Bion, not only the well-being of individuals but also the security and purposes, the systems and the structures of the groups to which they belong. In that we are changing and evolving as individuals and groups, life involves the re-shaping of identity from time to time. Our view of the world and our selves within it can change and when they do we experience loss and emotions associated with grief: anger, anxiety, and guilt, for example.[20] When we understand ourselves as persons affected by HIV, cumulative grief more intensely influences who we are, how we function, and how we relate. It will determine how we do theology.

A better understanding of the psycho-dynamic and psychoanalytic complexities of multiple losses and their emotional impact allows us to respond more sensitively to the challenges and opportunities of potential and real change as well as to any resistance to it.

Bion argues that all individuals and groups develop, consciously or unconsciously, strategies to accommodate the fears and anxieties inherent in all human experience. His identification of the strategies in terms of dependency, pairing, and fight/flight offers further insight into the roles of institutions and the responses of individuals and into aspects of change management.

In every group Bion finds the primitive anxieties about personal survival mingle with the need to further the task of the group. He demonstrates how societies, by institutionalizing appropriate receptacles for this emotional activity, seek to prevent anxieties from disabling or toppling social structures: for dependency anxieties, the Church; for fight/flight anxieties, the army; and for pairing/hope anxieties, the aristocracy. Each group presents both concrete models and metaphors for survival strategies.

Anxiety-arousing situations, and many exist in any life-span and in any HIV context, can awaken in each of us a memory or a fantasy about threats to our survival as an independent being. A failure to appreciate the abiding influence of early years experience, however unconscious, obscure, or vivid the memory, will limit, hinder, even confound choices when it impacts upon the present. According to Bion, for example, dependency which is acknowledged and appropriately accommodated, will benefit individuals, groups, and entire societies. The Church functions as a repository for dependency needs. But now the Church has AIDS.

Fears and anxieties over personal survival find expression in both combative and aggressive behavior and in withdrawal and escape. Anger, outrage, hate, and fear are the characteristic emotions of this assumption. Although Bion's fight/flight receptacle is the army, the concept will have increased significance to a Church which both outrages and is outraged by people affected by HIV. Internal and external targets and flight/fight strategies take shape. We withdraw from shared-cup communion, claim the high moral ground, close ranks, appeal to scripture, and create a God to authorize discrimination and injustice against people affected and infected with HIV. But now the army and the Church have HIV. The institutional roles become blurred and confused. Alertness to such projection, "the unwitting attribution to others of trends within a person's own personality," and the reverse, introjection, is necessary if in this HIV crisis scapegoating, ghettoizing, and guilt-induced self-denigration can be avoided at both corporate and individual levels. [21]

This institutional role confusion surfaces again in relation to memories and hope. For Bion, the pairing function of the aristocracy represents an attempt to ensure hoped-for survival. A Church which incorporates in its foundational myths divine/human alliances of the most intimate kind can fulfil a need for memory and hope. But can a Church with HIV fulfill that need? Or can an aristocracy with AIDS fulfill that need?

Bion's models, by connecting early life emotional responses with institutions, gives us a new way of understanding the Church and moves us into an appreciation of HIV's potentially massive impact on institutional and personal functioning and a better appreciation of the difficulties in responding to HIV solely as a health issue. Having offered Church and religion to foster or shelter dependency, the army to free us from our concern about fight/flight responses, and an aristocracy to provide the structures and the dynasties to keep alive our hopes for survival, a virus now challenges the functionality of these "container" models.

For if bishop, duke, and general each has AIDS, upon whom or what do we project our emotional responses to memoried evolutions? How do societies neutralize or make creative use of that intense, potentially destructive emotional pressure on individuals, partnerships, families, and communities when traditional and familiar options fail them? How do we understand self and world when every "diseased" penis, womb, and breast contradicts a world which has learned to base much of its self-understanding on the cognitive and moral optimism of Freudian and post-Freudian developmental theories of the human being?

The Church as institution will continue to fulfil its "Bion-ic" roles. In the responses to HIV during recent years, we already detect echoes of a medieval paradigm positing celibacy and asexuality as ideal responses to the world (then facing syphilis), responses which ultimately support a resurgence of dualistic patriarchal and reactionary trends and which are symptoms of crisis instead of mature responses.

However, any failure on the part of the Church to recognize the realities of its own HIV infection and the HIV infection of the world will hasten the destruction of both; and the Church will be put under increasing pressure to provide/be the general to lead the troops into battle or into retreat from a world with HIV (fight/flight), to provide/be the leader, whether person or idea, who ensures hope by never being born (pairing), and to provide/be the leader who will play "the role of magical god who can deliver the group from all ills."[22] In other words, the prospect becomes one of increased and increasing dogmatic, authoritarian intervention.

But what does this lifting into view of a new perspective on Church reveal about discerning reality? Only when the group/institution, like the infant, realizes that the roots of its anxiety lie within itself, that "the goodness and the badness is located within each individual," will the emotional force be neutralized and the reality be recognized and faced maturely. [23]

Only then will the pragmatic approach to preventing HIV infection, regarding HIV solely as a health issue, be understood as an increasingly urgent need. Public Health Medicine, with new allies, will continue to argue that infection is best prevented in person-affirming culturally appropriate programs and environments; pastoral instead of authoritarian. The urgency is reflected by the WHO's Global Program on AIDS:

> It is time to fight denial, discrimination, complacency, among governments, communities, and individuals. With no cure or vaccine in sight, prevention and education must remain absolute priorities.
>
> It is time to bridge the deepening resource gap....GPA calculates that 1.5-2.9 billion dollars per year needs to be spent on AIDS prevention in the developing world: 10-20 times the current sum.
>
> It is time to reduce the vulnerability of women to HIV infection by improving their health, their education, their economic prospects, and their legal and social status.
>
> It is time to provide the young people of this world with the knowledge and means to protect themselves from infection....
>
> It is time to set up strong prevention and education campaigns in the workplace....
>
> It is time to ensure that humane, dignified care for people with HIV and AIDS is available everywhere....[24]

5. Discerning Realities

Bion, drawing on the work of Melanie Klein, focuses attention on the interacting emotional forces within all groups and allows us to see that the psychological history of each individual impacts upon groups, organizations, and institutional social structures in profound ways. In a book first published in 1942, Erich

Fromm, pursuing a similar theme, states that "to understand the dynamics of social processes we must understand the dynamics of psychological operating within the individual."[25] However clearly prescribed and collectively subscribed are the group's aims and objectives, creedal and mission statements, what is likely is that the varying emotional and psychological needs and responses of any group's members will often be in conflict, creating problematic relationships and putting stress on structures.

More starkly put, where we seek to distance ourselves from parental, organizational, or institutional authority or structuring and feel frustrated, diminished, even dehumanized by them, another's sole goal is to lose herself/himself within them, be sheltered by them, even subject to them. This polarity of need lifts the institutional role into new light and exposes the dialogical tension inherent to any engagement with discerned realities, all of which are "correct."

The insights of psychology can illumine the impact of emotion upon Church as institution and as organization as well as, more familiarly, upon Church as individual. For only in the recognition and understanding of that emotional force can that Church as both counselor and counseled better discern itself and understand itself and its world; then the Church can better engage in dialogue with and respond to HIV and people affected by HIV.

The growing self-understanding results in the sometimes painful uncovering of hitherto hidden factors—unjust actions, dishonest certitude, perhaps—potentially damaging to both parties in the dialogical relationship. But, as Michael Jacobs argues, referring to the counselor as individual,

> through self-knowledge he will be less tempted to project his own difficulties on to the client and he will be less inclined to try and resolve them through another person.... His insight into himself will enhance his understanding of the other.[26]

In conclusion, we are bound to ask, how can the Church know itself more correctly when its members' fears and anxieties around HIV drive the "knowing" and can obstruct the process? How can the Church respond to and maturely manage its own and the world's HIV diagnosis? Mature discernment is the key to "correct" discernment. Indeed, one can argue that, ultimately, maturely discerning the realities of HIV will be a matter of survival, for that which presently offers hope for security may finally cost us the life it seeks to secure.

NOTES

1. S.C. Darby, D.W. Ewart, P.L.F. Giangrande, P.J. Dolin, C.R. Rizza, R.J.P. Spooner, "Morality Before and After HIV Infection in the Complete UK Population of Haemophiliacs," *Nature*, 377 (1995), pp. 79-82 (p. 79).

2. HIV and AIDS Treatments Directory, *National AIDS Manual* (London: National AIDS Manual Publications, 1995).

3. *Ibid.*, pp. 20-34.

4. *Ibid.*, p. 109.

5. *Ibid.*, pp. 130, 886. See also Panos, *World AIDS*, 34 (London: Panos, 1994), p. 12.

6. *Ibid.*, pp. 254-256.

7. Charles Perrow and Manro F. Guillan, *The AIDS Disaster* (New Haven: Yale University Press, 1990), pp. 131-151.

8. World Health Organisation, *World AIDS Day Newsletter* (Geneva: WHO Office of Information, 1990).

9. Panos, *Private Decision, Public Debate: Women, Reproduction, and Population* (London: Panos, 1994), p.5.

10. *Ibid.*, p.50.

11. Susan Sontag, *AIDS and Its Metaphors* (New York: Farrar, Straus and Giroux, 1989).

12. *Ibid.*, p. 25.

13. Thom Gunn, *The Man with Night Sweats* (London: Faber and Faber, 1992), p. 69.

14. Department of Health, *HIV/AIDS/Sexual Health and Britain's Faith Communities: A Special Health Alliance; Conference Report* (London: Department of Health, 1994), p. 38.

15. *Ibid.*, p. 39.

16. Michael Jacobs, *Swift to Hear* (London: SPCK, 1987), p. 21.

17. Michael Jacobs, *Still Small Voice* (London: SPCK, 1987), p. 35.

18. World Health Organization, *Guidelines for Counselling about HIV Infection and Disease* (Geneva: World Health Organization, 1990), p.12.

19. W. R. Bion, *Experiences in Groups and Other Papers* (London: Tavistock, 1968), p. 160.

20. See Martin Herbert, *Psychology for Social Workers* (Basingstoke: Macmillan, 1986), p. 278; John Bowlby, *Attachment and Loss*, Vol. 3 (London: Hogarth 1980), p. 40; and Elisabeth Kubler-Ross, *AIDS: The Ultimate Challenge* (New York: Collier Macmillan, 1987).

21. David M Wulff, *Psychology of Religion* (New York: Wiley, 1991), pp. 9-23.

22. Robert de Board, *The Psychoanalysis of Organizations* (London: Tavistock, 1978), p. 45.

23. *Ibid*, p. 47.

24. World Health Organization, *Global AIDS News* (Geneva: World Health Organization, 1993), p. 18.

25. Erich Fromm, *The Fear of Freedom* (London: Routledge and Kegan Paul, 1984), p. ix.

26. Jacobs, *Still Small Voice,* p. 48.

Ten

THE CATEGORY OF "PERSONHOOD" AND ACCESS TO HEALTH CARE

Matthew Bonzo

A grand tradition stands in which philosophers and theologians have argued about what separates persons from non-persons. The answers to the question "what makes a person a person?" have been varied. Is it the capability for being rational, is it possessing a highly evolved system of communications, or is it a purely biological distinction? Recently, this discussion has emerged with added significance and took on new implications in the area of health care. The distinction between persons and non-persons has entered the debate surrounding what criterion or criteria should be used to determine the level of health care that a given body should receive. The assumption of this discussion is that our ability to make the person/non-person distinction is foundational to our making the ethical choice or adequately justified decision regarding the funds/time/effort spent on any given patient.

The intent of my chapter is not to enter the conversation surrounding persons and health care by offering another argument for a different definition of personhood or personal identity which will lead us to make the right decision regarding the allocation of limited medical resources. Instead, I want to step back and question the assumption regarding the connection between our ability to distinguish theoretically person from non-person and to justify our ethical decisions.

This questioning will take place in two parts. First, I will summarize a recent article in the medical ethics literature which uses the person/non-person distinction as a basis for making some types of medical decisions. The article will be used to highlight the concomitant privileging of one group over the other when the person/non-person distinction is made. Second, I will consider the unwarranted priority granted to persons over non-persons in any attempt to define person in terms of a distinctive set of abilities or characteristics. The implicit preferencing of sameness in the person/non-person distinction attempts to limit the ambiguity of life at the cost of denying otherness. The ambiguity present when such a conception of ethics is questioned does not mean the end of making decisions, but places ethical (including bioethical) decisions in a context of undecidability. The exposure of the implicit privileging in the person/non-person distinction to a context of undecidability allows a less violent relationship to evolve between care-giver and the cared-for as together we suffer with our decisions.

1. Persons and Non-Persons

While several illustrations of the foundational nature of the person/non-person distinction for medical ethics exist in the burgeoning literature of the field, an excellent example is Dan Brock's article, "Justice and the Severely Demented Elderly." Brock's concern in this article is the allocation of resources in cases where elderly persons who suffer from severe cases of dementia are involved. However, in the process of developing his guidelines for deciding the amount of resources due to the patient with severe dementia, he reveals his criterion for making the distinction between person and non-person.

As Brock has noted, once he has established this basic distinction, several health care allocation decisions can readily be made. Brock suggests his criterion for being a person when he states that "the effects of dementia that are my special concern here are the erosion of memory and other cognitive functions that attack and...ultimately destroy personal identity and personhood in the patient."[1] While personhood is not equated with personal identity, both are intimately connected with the human capabilities of memory and higher cognitive functions. Brock is not making the person/non-person distinction based on whether the body is conscious or irreversibly unconscious. The distinction is taking place at a different level. Brock argues that when "the crucial role played by memory and other forms of psychological continuity" ceases to function adequately, a loss of personal identity results.[2] Without the psychological ability to establish and maintain a sense of self identity, a person ceases to exist. The loss of the so-called higher functions of the brain means a person has become a non-person.

Brock considers the Permanently Vegetative State (PVS) patient and the severely demented patient as examples where the person/non-person distinction is helpful. The aim of medicine, which Brock defines as "the promotion of opportunity through the prevention or treatment of disability" is no longer possible in a PVS patient because "opportunity presupposes capacities for agency and action."[3] Brock argues that if you use any philosophical understanding of personhood, including the two major philosophical traditions of physical continuity and psychological continuity, the PVS patient falls short of meeting the definition. Inevitably, the PVS patient falls into the category of non-person. With being accorded the status of non-person, the PVS patient places less of a demand on us for health care resources.

While Brock assumes that the distinction between person and non-person can be drawn in the case of PVS patients, he sees a little more difficulty in applying the categorization to patients with severe dementia. Because patients with severe dementia still have conscious experience and are capable of limited agency, the demarcation between person and non-person would seem to be more clouded. As previously mentioned, Brock does maintain a distinction between personhood and personal identity—one which carries implications for his consideration of a patient with severe dementia. While someone with dementia may not be able psychologically to sustain a personal identity, one could continue to have qualities which could qualify one as a person. In some schemata, the loss of identity does not necessarily mean the loss of personhood. The demented patient could meet designated minimal criteria for personhood even though the ability to identify oneself may be lost.

Though Brock, too, does not want a conflation of personhood and personal identity, he does posit a close interconnection between the two. This interconnection can be seen in Brock's definition of personhood given in terms of memory and cognitive capabilities. In the case of dementia, Brock explains that the patient's "cognitive capacities and, in particular, memory are so destroyed as to eliminate the psychological continuity and connectedness."[4] He argues that without the continuity (identity) sustained by memory, a difficulty arises in according the patient with severely limited cognitive capabilities the status of person. For Brock, the loss of identity ruthlessly impinges upon one's personhood. Though the patient with dementia's loss of the abilities which make one a person is not quite as obvious as the PVS patient's loss of personhood, Brock's connection of identity with personhood allows him to place the patient with severe dementia in the same category of non-person.

Being considered a non-person, or to use Brock's term, "a non-human being," is not equated with the cessation of all physical functions. A living body does elicit some caring response from a care-giver. However, the obligations experienced are not as great as those we have toward a full-fledged person. Brock presents this gradation of obligation by talking about two types (stages?) of death: the death of the person and the death of the human being. He argues that the difference between a loss of a designated set of capabilities and the absence of all bodily functioning "warrants distinguishing between the death of the person (so-called higher brain death) and the death of the human being (so-called whole brain death)."[5] With this distinction, the argument can be made that ceasing to be a person is not the same as being declared clinically dead. Brock, adopting the whole-brain-death criterion, says that in a dead human being all brain activity, including the brain stem, has perished. For the death of the person, higher brain-functions like memory will have ceased. The category of non-person is for those who fall short of meeting the criteria for personhood while still unfortunately having some minimal bodily functioning. So we now have a third category in which *homo sapiens* can be placed between being a person and being dead.

I will briefly give an enumeration of the categories. The most privileged group is persons. The criterion to be included is higher brain-function which incorporates memory and some cognitive abilities. The second group is human beings in which one must have lower brain-functioning to be included. The final group includes the dead who have no brain-function and probably are not too upset about being the least privileged group. From this basic categorization, Brock argues for a designated level of access to health care resources for each level. Persons, as the most valued beings, have the greatest access to health care because of the importance of their status. As for the brain-dead, Brock acknowledges that little argument from any side can be advanced for continued allocation of any type of health-care resources.

The crux of Brock's argument lies in the second classification. Mere human beings as non-persons do not obligate us in the same way that persons do. Their less privileged status accords them less access to limited resources. To reiterate, Brock's position does not demand that non-persons be abandoned. Instead, the category of non-person is argued by Brock as the means to a fairer division of limited health care resources. By limiting access to non-persons, who are a group of patients who in the past have had an equal, if not greater, access, Brock advances an across-the-board standard for the future, just division of medical care. Because the PVS patients and patients with severe dementia do not meet the criteria of being a person, they should obligate us in a lesser manner, requiring only palliative care.

2. Persons as Theoretical Abstractions

The work of Brock and other medical ethics experts on the person/non-person distinction is motivated by a real concern which plays a more prominent role in making treatment decisions as we are forced to recognize the inevitability of some type of medical rationing. My intent is not to deny that the difficult decisions involved in the distribution of resources must be made. Instead, the fear and trembling with which we must approach the choice to withhold medical treatments from a given individual or group is the cause of my apprehension.

The person/non-person distinction attempts to ease our pain in making these decisions by giving us a hierarchy of obligations which provides a ready made comfort through drawing the boundaries for our compassion. The overcoming of ambiguity in bioethical decisions is sought by abstracting qualities or functions of human beings in order to limit those who can be granted the status of person. The place granted a given individual in the hierarchy determines the level of health care she or he will receive. In this prioritizing of one set of qualities or functions, one group is privileged and set over against those who are excluded. The criterion for being admitted to the privileged group is sameness; that is, those in the privileged group share the same qualities or capabilities. Those with a different set of qualities/functions are placed outside the group and considered of lesser status. Brock's person/non-person distinction is a stark example of an ethics of exclusion which has been at the forefront of the postmodernist critique of ethics.

While for some postmodern philosophers, speaking of persons or personhood already shows an inability to distance oneself from the logic of exclusion, I still want to speak of being a person. But I do not want to speak about persons by offering another list of defining characteristics. Instead, I prefer to speak of persons as we experience them. I do not think we have much of a problem deciding whether the things we meet are persons. Some philosophers speculate about robots and the like, but in our day-to-day existence, we know when we meet persons, whether they are sick or healthy, rational or irrational. We primarily encounter them not as theoretical constructs but as living, breathing bodies that eat, reproduce, laugh, cry, and engage other activities. I am not saying that the person is the sum of these practices, but this is how we meet them.

To reduce human life to one of these activities and prioritize it as the defining characteristic necessarily denies most of the person we encounter. Human life resists any attempt to define the self by absolutizing a given aspect of its being, such as its biological, economical, or rational dimensions. Human life is multidimensional, and the value of being human cannot be contained or explained by only one dimension. As such, a person cannot be reduced to a concept or set of concepts which understand the richness of human life only in terms of centered modal metaphors. The centering of any dimension of human existence can be helpful in explaining part of who we are, but it does so at the cost of blurring the totality. To take one dimension or a set of dimensions as being the essential person necessarily excludes those in whom a lack of the listed capabilities are present, or in which the capabilities are severely diminished. Human life's resistance to being reduced to one dimension or a set of dimensions points to the primary grasping of me by the person, instead of my objectifying of the other through abstractions.

3. Beyond Medical Ethics

In the grand tradition, anxiety naturally arises when the theoretical foundation for making the distinction between persons and non-persons trembles before the other. Without the primacy of our foundations, our ability to make ethical decisions in the tradition is severely limited. Without such a foundation, the fear arises that anything goes as "person" becomes an arbitrary category that we will be unable to enact because we lack the assurance that our actions are universally justified. But these options are only realizable if persons are equated with the theoretical constructions about persons.

John Caputo has argued that the loss of foundations does not result in either arbitrary relativism or paralyzing fear. Caputo maintains that his critique of foundations, of which I understand Brock's attempt at a person/non-person distinction to be a type, does not opt for non-action. The search for certainty has had a propensity for covering the original difficulty of life. The decisions established through this logic of certainty must be exposed as pseudo-actions. Because foundations pre-determine what path to follow, decisions are always already made. Only when the excluded other strips away the pretension of certainty can real decisions be made.

The revelation of the ambiguity of life "does not leave action behind, does not let us enter a new world, make a leap into a different sphere where there is no longer any need to act." We must still act, but without "the security of metaphysical foundations."[6] Caputo later says of our situation, "we act because something has to be done."[7] Yet this something to be done has no unshakeable ground on which we can justify doing it. Instead, we "tak[e] what action seems wise, and not without misgivings."[8] We no longer have a law which orders our actions and relationships with one another. This loss of metaphysical first principles does not result in chaos, anarchy, and closed selves becoming laws unto themselves. For even after ethics, the other still grasps me. Though we cannot account for it theoretically, Caputo asserts that "obligation happens."[9]

The obligation which happens between a person and an other points to the web of relations in which a person is enmeshed. By obligation, Caputo means

> a superficial-horizontal communication between one human being and another, a certain line of force that runs along the surface upon which you and I stand: the obligation I have to you (and you to me, but this is different) and the both of 'us' to 'others.'[10]

Persons exist in relationships, and when we consider our relationships we realize we are bound to the other. We do not consent, contract, or agree to this obligation. Obligation seizes me. And since I must still act, my action takes place within the context of my obligation, and my relationship to others. The ability to distinguish person from non-person is not foundational to being obliged. My obligation to the other is not rooted in her ability to meet my standards. We are always already obligated to the other. This obligation is not lost because the other fails to conform to my theoretical expectations. The other shatters my expectations of sameness and breaks through to grasp me.

Brock's person/non-person distinction is an attempt at establishing a first principle in order to calm the flux of life. From his basis, decisions come more easily. But Brock's privileging of one group over another is prejudicial and cannot be ultimately justified. The loss of the person/non-person distinction to make our distribution of resources decisions ethical does not result in either a paralysis of inaction or excessive arbitrariness. We are still obliged to the other, no matter what their set of abilities or functions.

The result of the loss of person/non-person distinction is the sting of the flux as the difficulty of making decisions is accepted instead of denied. No longer does a pre-determined hierarchy of obligations exist into which we slot the other. Instead, a recognition exists of the complicated web of multi-level, intertwining obligations to the other or others in which we live. This tangled web is further complicated by our limited resources. We cannot meet every obligation. Our situation demands a differentiated allocation of reserves. But the allocation always takes place within the web of obligation to the other or others which prohibits either a dismissal or lessening of status. This is the ambiguity of life which makes our decisions undecidable. Nevertheless we must decide. Obligation toward the other always already relativizes the "rightness" of any choice we do make. It prevents us from declaring any choice which privileges one obligation over another obligation as being justifiable.

Though ethical decisions may not be ultimately justifiable, the web of obligation prevents the decisions from being arbitrary. The sorting of obligations calls upon wisdom. I do not want to spend much time defining wisdom. Following Caputo, by wisdom I do not mean the establishment of a theoretical calculus whereby we plug in the variables and get the answer. Wisdom is learning to live, to understand what kind of fruit is born by a variety of decisions. In the health-care sphere, I take it that being wise would mean the decisions about given cases should be based on information complete as possible regarding things like: prognosis, cost, comparison to similar cases, honest medical judgment, and prediction. Brock and I could agree on the type of care a given patient with dementia should receive. But the decision should not be arrived at because it has been (pre)determined the patient is less than a person and, therefore, has less privileged access to health care. A lower level of treatment may be chosen because in the mess of sorting obligations, we had to choose. Along what Callahan has called "the ragged edge," the consequences of such a decision are hard to live with.[11] No comfort is taken in making such decisions, yet perhaps it is the only way of coping with the difficulty of life.

4. Conclusion

This chapter took on a new meaning for me with the recent death of my mother-in-law from cancer. With the onset of cancer, inevitable decisions have to be faced. Maybe it would be easy if a simple formula existed which solved the problems inherent in making difficult choices. Yet I not only question a particular approach to answering the dilemmas of health care ethics. More than critiquing a given method, I doubt the existence of first principles from which the justness of any action can be deduced which would be necessary for such a method. Terms like "morally justified" and "distributive justice" disguise the prejudicial privileging of one group over another in differentiations like Brock's person/non-person distinction by appearing to be the only acceptable way. The ambiguity of life relativizes these answers, even in the realm of health care ethics. We cannot overcome the obligation from each person we encounter. Yet, the overabundance of obligations takes place in a context of limited resources. This conundrum does not preclude action, for we must act, even if we have lost the assurances which metaphysical foundations granted us. The field of health care ethics is one of the more explicit examples of a realm in which we must act even though our webs of obligations relativize every decision. Not to act would be disastrous. Our inability to escape the flux of life means we must dirty our hands with many complicating factors including economic and political concerns. Sorting obligations as a community means an open discussion instead of the closed monologue typical of established policy.

NOTES

1. Dan Brock, "Justice and the Severely Demented Elderly," *Journal of Medicine and Philosophy*, 13 (February 1988), pp. 73-99.

2. *Ibid.*, p. 74.

3. *Ibid.*, p. 79.

4. *Ibid.*, p. 85.

5. *Ibid.*

6. John Caputo, *Radical Hermeneutics* (Bloomington, Ind.: Indiana University Press, 1993), p. 239.

7. *Ibid.*, p. 240.

8. *Ibid.*, p. 239. Brackets mine.

9. John Caputo, *Against Ethics* (Bloomington, Ind.: Indiana University Press, 1993), p. 6.

10. *Ibid.*, p. 5.

11. Daniel Callahan, *What Kind of Life?* (New York: Simon and Schuster, 1990).

Eleven

BRAIN TRANSPLANTS AND THE ORTHODOX VIEW OF PERSONHOOD

Gavin J. Fairbairn

The view that some human individuals are not people is useful to many of those who engage, professionally or philosophically, with numerous distressing situations that arise in the lives that people lead, or who find themselves bound up personally in such situations. For example, it is useful at the beginning of life when it may be used to deny not only personhood but life, to small human beings—usually those who are disabled or in some way inconvenient for bigger folks.

In this chapter, I am concerned with the way in which some people— those that I shall refer to as "orthodox personists"—divide small human beings into two groups—those who qualify for the plaudit "person" and those who do not, and who use this division as a way of deciding which babies should live, and which should die. Not only may small people be separated into people and non-people; as has happened at several points in history, big people now exist whose personhood may be denied and who may be denied life as a consequence. As a result of brain injury or disease, human individuals at a later stage in their lives may enter into a phase of their biological existence that would lead some others to exclude them from the category "person" while acknowledging that the case that they were once persons is unequivocal. The most public examples of situations in which the personhood of human individuals who are past babyhood is denied, arise in relation to discussions about the status of people in a so-called "persistent vegetative state" (PVS). Those who become involved in such discussions sometimes invoke the notion not only that such individuals are not the person "they once were" but that they have ceased to be a person of any kind at all. The public discussion of such cases has become more and more common in recent years. However, more frequently the case is that small disabled people, especially those that have yet to be born, will be regarded as non-persons. What is instructive is to reflect on the reasons that the personhood of little people is more often denied than that of big people; as a result they are often killed or "allowed to die"; for example, doing so casts light on medical decisions in relation to severely disabled neonates.[1]

1. Four Views of Personhood

In the matter of personhood four main possibilities emerge:

1. All and only human beings are people.

2. All but perhaps not only human beings are people.

3. Not all and not only human beings are people.

4. Not all but only human beings are people.

Of these, belief 1, (the belief that the only people who exist, are human people and that all existing human beings are people), is perhaps closest to what most people believe who have grown up to consider "human" and "person" as synonymous expressions that refer to members of the human species. By contrast, belief 3, is furthest from this, accepting as it does, both the possibility that you could have human beings who are not people and the possibility that there could be people who are not human beings. Like belief 3, belief 4 raises the possibility that human non-persons may exist; usually those human beings who are said not to be people are unwanted or undesirable—including, for example, severely disabled neonates and unwanted babies, disabled or not, before they are born. However, whereas belief 3 raises the possibility that people who are not human beings might exist, belief 4 assumes that only human beings can be persons.

Those who hold belief 2, like those who hold belief 1, are conservative on the question of whether human beings who are not people might exist, but by contrast to those who hold belief 1, those who hold to belief 2 believe that they are, or might be, non-human persons.

Belief 2 (the belief that all but perhaps not only human beings are people), is the view to which I hold personally as a matter of principle. Part of the reason is that I can see no distinction between human beings at different stages in their lives as human beings that would justify including some into the category "person" while excluding others.

Because I want to draw stark attention to my belief that human beings are people from the outset of their distinctively human lives, I choose to refer (some would argue question-beggingly) to young human individuals—babies and fetuses and embryos—as "small people." I would also use the expression to refer to small people of other species, should there be any. Interestingly, those who would accuse me of question-begging when I refer to small people as people, are themselves often guilty of question-begging. They are guilty of question-begging because they hijack the concept of the person, then they justify the use to which they put it by begging the question of whether "person" is amenable of definition. Then by offering a definition which excludes certain individuals from the category of persons they manage (by their account of the value of lives and of individuals), to justify the killing of such individuals, allowing them to die or treating them as if they are dead.

2. The Orthodox View of Personhood

The denial of personhood to some human individuals begins with the belief that as a result of immaturity, brain injury, or disease, such individuals may not display characteristics which have been arbitrarily decided are necessary for personhood. Many variations arise on the claim that criteria can be delineated by which we may measure claims to personhood on behalf of individuals—variations, for example, about the characteristics that are said to be necessary for personhood and also about the extent to which these have to be displayed. However, the overlap between the views of those whose work has gone to create the common notion that people are only people and, in particular human people are only people, if they pass some test based on lists of criteria, is such that I have to come to think of them as comprising a kind of orthodoxy which I refer to as the "orthodox view of persons." I do not intend to argue for the existence of this orthodox view which is found in the work of philosophers such as Peter Singer, Helga Kuhse, and John Harris.[2]

Orthodox personists do not believe that being a human being and being a person are the same thing. They do not believe (or at any rate they tend to claim that they do not believe) that being human is especially significant, morally speaking. Orthodox personists, and others who embrace the orthodox view of personhood (instead of a single, unitary view, it would, I suppose, be more correct to refer to a family of such views), believe that what makes people significant, is that they have certain characteristics, including for example, self-consciousness, the ability to use language, to entertain plans for the future and to remember the past. They believe that the possession of such characteristics is what makes people people, that those who would be people, who will be people, are not people unless and until they have developed them.

Proponents of the orthodox view have different opinions about what characteristics are most significant; and usually they are ambiguous about which or even how many characteristics an individual must display in order to be a person. In other words, instead of specifying individual characteristics that are necessary for personhood, they offer a list of characteristics some number of which, taken together, indicate that what we have is a person and not something that, for example, just looks like a person.

Lists of characteristics whose presence is thought significant in admitting an individual into the category of persons and whose absence is thought significant in the decision to exclude them from this category, often include characteristics of distinct kinds: that is, they may contain both physiological and psychological characteristics. Psychological features that are often mentioned include the presence of experiences and mental activities such as self awareness, remembering the past and laying plans for the future, reasoning (at whatever level is thought necessary), and for language use. But sometimes the physical potential for psychological features of this kind is what is thought to define personhood—or minimally, the possibility of personhood, instead of the psychological characteristics themselves. And so, for example, features such as the presence of a fully functioning brain or cerebral cortex are at times thought sufficient for the possibility of personhood.

However, although no universal set of characteristics exists about which all orthodox personists agree, self consciousness (or the capability for self-consciousness of a minimal kind) is often considered to be the single most significant feature that must be present in order for an individual to qualify for the plaudit "person."

I do not intend to offer a lengthy critique of the orthodox view. However, I want to draw attention to the arbitrary way in which the characteristics thought to be definitive of personhood are selected, some unspecified number of which an individual must display, in order to be given the respect and care normally shown to persons. The idea that a cluster of characteristics can be delineated by which we may tell which individuals are persons and which are not, involves giving the construct "person" the appearance of objectivity, almost as if we are dealing with a biological category like "*homo sapiens*." This is useful when it comes to making decisions between people, say in medicine. Those who adopt a view of persons which permits apparently objective decisions about which human beings are, and which are not persons, have at their disposal a convenient and apparently straightforward way of deciding, for example, who should benefit from health-care resources or who should have their needs treated preferentially. They can say in an apparently objective and almost scientific way "This is a person and that is not, therefore we should give the resource to this and not that." The moral convenience of such a view of personhood has much to commend it in psychological terms—it takes away the necessity for soul searching and balancing the claims of those whose lives are being weighed against one another. However, its convenience does not make it morally correct.

How then does the orthodox philosopher decide which characteristics are to be taken as definitive of personhood? The procedure is simple. We look at paradigm cases of persons—folk, say, like you and me, and decide what about us is valuable, what characteristics make us worthy of special respect—whether in ourselves or because we support other characteristics. In doing so, we attempt to make a judgement about what is valuable about us not just to ourself, but to everyone. These characteristics are then said to be the defining characteristics of personhood—those who display them are said to be persons while those who do not display them are not.

Since those who adopt the orthodox view of personhood wish to argue that the killing of some humans or allowing them to die is morally permissible, what is not surprising is to find that the characteristics they choose as indicators of personhood usually exclude such individuals. So, for example, they might choose characteristics that will allow human embryos, fetuses, and neonates to be killed (or, and this is more usual in the case of neonates, "allowed to die"), when they are unwanted, say because of a disability or because they are otherwise inconvenient.

Now I confess to agreeing that characteristics of the kind cited by orthodox personists make the class of persons different from other individuals such as cats, dogs, goldfish, trees, and personal computers, and I acknowledge that such characteristics in people are especially valued. However, I do not agree that these characteristics are what makes people valuable. I may value an ingot of platinum because it sparkles nicely in the sunshine but it is not its sparkling alone that gives it value. No reason exists at all to say that displaying one or more of the set of characteristics that we value in human persons is what makes a person, a person. This would be like saying that because we value green apples for their greenness, crunchiness, and bitter sweetness, what makes them green apples is their greenness, bitter sweetness, and crunchiness; and if what makes green apples green apples are these characteristics, then peas, conference pears, decent celery, and lime lollipops are also members of the class of green apples; indeed, anything else which shared one or more of these characteristics would by such a line of reasoning be a green apple.

Nor do I agree that human beings who do not display the characteristics that we highly value in people may be treated differently from those who do, just because they are not yet displaying them, or even because they are unlikely ever to display them. And I do not agree that because they are not displaying such characteristics, these people are not people.

3. "All but perhaps not only Human Beings are People"

In spite of what orthodox personists—both modern and not so modern have to say, our concept "person" gains its identity and focus from the group of individuals to whom we generally apply the term—that is, from the group of human individuals with whom and in relation to whom, we make our lives—intellectual, social, and moral. Although unborn, human fetuses, embryos, call them what you will, are unequivocally part of the human species and therefore part of the group in relation to whom the concept "person" has gained its meaning. For this reason, I can see no reason to exclude them from the category "person" but every reason to include them. Since no non-arbitrary stage can be pointed to in the development of human beings at which they become people, the sensible and I believe morally correct thing to do, is to regard them as people as soon as fertilization is completed and perhaps because of the difficulty in pinpointing this time exactly, from some time shortly before. Basing our relationships with and acts towards them on this means that should it turn out that I am mistaken and that human beings turn into people at some time during their gestational lives, instead of always being people, we will have treated some individuals who are not people as if they were. However, this seems less morally reprehensible than taking the risk of treating some people as if they are not.

I am thus conservative on the question of whether some humans might not be people. However, I am less conservative on the question of whether people who are not human beings might exist. I am less conservative on this because I acknowledge the possibility that we might recognize in a non-human species or life form, just those things that make human persons similar to one another and different from non-persons. And thus I wish to remain agnostic on the question of whether, in addition to the group of human persons in relation to whom our concept "person" has developed and in relation to whom it has its central use, people exist who are non-human. Indeed, I would be pleased to hear from anyone who reads this chapter, who has come across non-human people of any other species—from this planet or any other; and I would be especially keen to hear from anyone who is himself or herself, a non-human person. Incidentally, if and when persons of other species come to light, I believe we should take as much care of their embryos, fetuses, and babies as we do of human embryos, fetuses, and babies; I should hate to be thought speciesist.

4. Brain Transplants and the Concept of a Person

Perhaps like me, you entertain the possibility that somewhere in the universe there might be people who are not human people like us (I am assuming now that like me, you are a human person). Perhaps like me, you entertain the possibility that people of other species live close by—that is, for example, that some animals such as apes and whales and so on, might be people. Perhaps like me, you watched a program on UK television years ago, about work with chimpanzees (BBC, August 1993) in which chimps were shown engaging in numerous activities which made it difficult to avoid considering the possibility that they are people like us—dimmer perhaps, but people nonetheless.

For example, we saw a chimp who was able, from a large array of photographs, to match objects that he was informed about verbally. We saw chimps communicating not only through human based sign language but using a concept keyboard through which, by pressing appropriate symbols, they could communicate in human speech through a digitized voice box. Another chimp could perform simple mathematical tasks such as matching numerals (up to 9) to groups of objects and distinguishing which of two amounts (up to 9) of sweets was the larger; this chimp could also choose from two numerals the one that represented the larger number of sweets. One chimp when asked to do so could follow complex commands such as "Fetch a Coca Cola for X" even when the Coca Cola was in a fridge in another room; another used the concept keyboard to ask his human companion to take him somewhere (to "ape farm"), though getting there involved a journey in a vehicle.

Recently, I have been working with thought experiments similar to those of eminent human philosophers like Bernard Williams and Derek Parfit, in which the brains of human individuals are swapped around, though some of what I have been thinking about involves the possibility of interspecies mixing of brains.[3] In the first of these, I have found myself wondering whether, if we were able successfully to transplant a baby chimp's brain into a human baby whose own brain was either absent or non-functioning, we would have a chimp in a human baby body? Or would we have a human baby with a chimp's brain? Questions similar to this and others that follow, might also be asked in relation to interspecies brain transplants between human babies and babies of other higher apes, for example, orangutan babies or gorilla babies.

If a human being, the baby would be a human being with more possibility for intelligent behavior than before because the baby's brain, though non-human, would be fully functioning. If a chimp, the baby would be a chimp who, growing up in possession of a human body, would have the possibility of doing the things that human bodies can do. The most significant of these is probably that because the baby now had a human voice box, the baby might be able to learn to speak like a human being. As a result of this and perhaps because people would react to the baby differently because of the human form, the baby might well become brighter than chimps are meant to become; consequently our chimp might develop and begin to display more of the characteristics that are often thought to define persons than we would normally expect of chimps. Support for the notion that a chimp occupying a human body might be treated differently than a chimp in a chimp body and hence might become brighter than he would have been otherwise, may be gained by considering some research with children with Down's Syndrome.

In the work in question, facial surgery was carried out on children with Down's partly in order to correct difficulties with large and labile tongues, and the problems that they cause in terms of the development of speech, but partly also to make cosmetic "improvements" to the appearance of the youngsters. Significantly, following surgery, it was reported that the children became brighter. We can easily hazard a guess at the reason for this; for example, given that after surgery they looked more "normal," it might be that people treated children who had received such surgery with expectations that were not limited and limiting in the way that they would most likely have done had their appearance been "typically Down's." As a result, the children in question were probably facilitated more in their intellectual development than they would have been had they maintained their Down's features.

So would our child be a human person with a chimp brain, or instead a chimp person living his life in a human body? Or would the baby instead be no kind of person at all but only a messed-up kind of chimpanzee living in a human body?

The question arises whether a capability for mental, social, and physical behaviors of a kind that depend upon a highly developed brain such as that possessed by most human beings, does determine personhood as many human people seem to suppose. Or perhaps rather, it is our relationship with God, in which case whether a human body with a chimp's brain was a person would not only depend upon God's relationship with humankind but also upon God's relationship with chimpkind.

5. Two Needy Babies

Turning to more weighty matters, I want now to share some of what I have been thinking about the possibility of brain transplants among small human beings.

Suppose that however gruesome the possibility, and whatever the ethical problems that arose during the experimental period, brain transplants have been perfected; suppose also that whereas it has been happening for a great many years, heart transplant surgery has continued to have a low level of success. Suppose, finally, that in a hospital known for its pioneering work in transplant procedures, two sets of parents have tragic life stories which come together in the following way.

Scene 1

> The Joneses baby was born after a normal pregnancy. Shortly after birth, however, a pediatrician discovers that baby Jones is suffering from a major and untreatable heart defect that will prove fatal. Though the success rate with such small people is low, his physicians decide that it would be worthwhile attempting a heart transplant if a suitable donor can be found; though they are aware that the chances of success are low, his parents, who are devastated by their baby's condition, are only too happy that attempts should be made to find a suitable donor.
>
> By chance, just as the doctors are discussing the question of transplants with Mr. and Mrs. Jones, another woman, Mrs. McDermott, is giving birth close by in the maternity ward. Whereas her baby has a perfectly sound heart, he is anencephalic, with all but his brain stem missing.

And so we have two sets of anxious and bereaved parents in Titworth Hospital on the day our story begins. Firstly the Jones, who are preparing themselves at best for the wait until a new heart can be found for their baby, or at worst for the grief and pain that they will feel if the search is unsuccessful; and, secondly, the

McDermotts, who are grieving for the complete baby that they had hoped for and facing with dread the almost inevitable early death of their child.

Scene 2

> News spreads quickly in Titworth Hospital and the doctors who are caring for baby J soon hear of the birth of baby M. Though realizing the devastating grief it must be causing his parents, they consider the news of baby M's birth and condition to be a piece of luck because they believe that being devoid of a brain he has no need for a heart. And so within minutes of hearing about his birth they seek out the doctors who are caring for him to request that his parents be asked to allow their child's heart to be used in order that they can save their patient, baby J. Furthermore, though they have no potential recipient in mind, they propose that the McDermotts should also be asked to make available other organs such as liver, kidneys and so on from their child, in order that other needy individuals might also be helped. They reason that since apart from the absence of a brain, baby M is in good condition, he represents a valuable resource for the medical community and it would be morally wrong not to do what they can to persuade his parents to permit the harvesting of his organs and the good that could be done with them.

Baby J's doctors are disappointed and surprised to discover that their request to be allowed to use baby M's heart to save baby J does not meet with immediate approval; and they are more surprised to discover why. It is not that baby M's doctors believe that his parents should be given time to recover from the shock and disappointment of realizing that their hopes for a complete if not perfect baby have been dashed, before being asked for permission to use their child as a donor—though they do believe this. Instead, they have another proposal in mind, which they put to baby J's doctors. Instead of their patient's heart being used to save baby J, they suggest, surely it would make more sense to use baby J's brain to save baby M. Their rationale for this proposal is that since brain transplants are perfected while heart transplants are not, the procedure with the greatest chance of success is the brain transplant. Transplanting baby J's brain into baby M's body, they argue, will ensure the survival of one child, whereas transplanting baby M's heart into baby J would be likely to end in the early death not only of the donor, but of the recipient.

Suppose that after hearing the moral and logical arguments in its favor, baby J's doctors were persuaded that the best outcome in this sorry situation was likely to be achieved if their patient's brain was transplanted into baby M's body, instead of baby M's heart being transferred into their patient's body. Suppose further that after considerable and understandable diffidence, baby J's parents were persuaded that giving up their baby's brain was for the best. They might, for example, have been persuaded by the argument that his brief life could gain meaning by giving life to another baby or babies who would otherwise have died. The doctors trying to persuade them of this might have said things of this kind: "Of course, you will still mourn; that is to be expected. But you would have the satisfaction of knowing that you had helped another child or children and another couple or couples to be happy." Feeling glad that their baby's death has meaning because it has allowed some other child to live is just what the parents of anencelphalic babies who give permission for their children to be used as donors are supposed to feel afterwards.

Scene 3

> The Jones give permission for their child's brain to be transplanted in order to save baby M. The operation is carried out successfully and the Jones mourn the death of their baby, taking what comfort they can in the new life their sacrifice has given to baby M, and the joy it has brought to his parents. Some weeks later the McDermotts leave the hospital pleased with life and carrying their new baby, complete with new brain and a fabricated top to his skull.

So within a small space of time two tragic stories have come together. One set of parents has agreed to allow the brain with which their baby was born, to be transferred to the body of a child born with little or no brain, because by doing so they could ensure that someone else can return home with a baby that they expect to survive. And another set of parents has gratefully benefited from the sacrifice that these generous others were prepared to make and as a result they are looking forward to seeing their child grow up.

But suppose that after some reflection the Jones's began to believe that instead of their baby having been used as a donor in a transplant performed to save baby M, the procedure that the doctors performed should be thought of as a body transplant in which their baby was saved using the now deceased baby M's body. In other words, suppose that in the end they came to believe that instead of being a McDermott, the baby that emerged from the operating theater was really a Jones, was really their baby. Would the Jones's be right coming to this conclusion?

The questions we have to settle are these:

> Are the McDermotts correct in thinking that the child that they brought home from hospital and for whom they have been caring, is their baby?
>
> Or is it a Jones, as the Joneses suppose?

Let's examine the line of reasoning the Joneses might have followed in coming to the conclusion that they have been grieving to no purpose because, though at the time of the transplant they thought he had died, their baby is alive and well in a new body, living with the McDermotts.

The Joneses' new belief draws upon the idea that a person is somehow intimately connected to that part of the body known as the brain—the bit that does the thinking, the experiencing, the feeling for us. The view that the brain is especially significant has some immediate and intuitive appeal; many people if asked to indicate where they think the "I" that feels and thinks and wants and so on, is located—will point to their heads and say something like, "In here," or, perhaps, "I'm here, just behind my eyes."

What, other than intuition, might make us agree with the Joneses' radical change of mind about the nature of the procedure in which their baby was involved either as a recipient or donor? We might do so if we embraced some version of the "orthodox" view of personhood which I have already discussed.

As I have pointed out, those who incline toward a version of the orthodox view, frequently argue that a human being cannot be a person unless among other things, one has a fully functioning brain—that allows one to think and remember, plan, reflect, use language, and be aware of one's existence. As a result, orthodox personists should agree with the Joneses' view that baby M could not, at birth, have been a person because, lacking a brain, the baby lacked the necessary physical substrate for these things; if a person is only a person if one demonstrates characteristics that require a functioning brain, the newly-born baby M in the absence of a brain, could not possibly have been a person, and could not even have had the potential of becoming a person. So at first sight, it looks as though the Joneses might gain the support of orthodox personists for their view that the operation to join together their baby's brain and baby M's body, should be thought of as a body transplant for their child who is now living as a McDermott.

But things are not so simple. Although for the sake of safety orthodox personists sometimes admit the possibility that those with the physical capability for the characteristics they have arbitrarily decided are necessary for personhood may, in a rudimentary way, be persons, the elasticity of the orthodox view is such that those who adhere to it most often maintain that it is only after an individual is displaying, or is capable of displaying, such characteristics, that he or she is a person. Those who have the potential to display these characteristics but who do not display them, are not persons according to this view but only potential persons, or "pre-persons." As a result, they are thought to warrant respect of the kind that is thought appropriate toward people.

So although at birth baby M was not, according to the orthodox view, a person, the same view would suggest that at birth baby J could not have been one either. Thus, though initially plausible because of the intuitive feeling that personhood is somehow intimately connected with our brain, orthodox personists would in the end have to disagree with the Joneses' interpretation of the physical facts, because somehow it may be silly to think that at birth baby J's brain had begun to be sufficiently "programmed" to allow them to think of it as housing a person. In other words, at the time that it was transplanted into baby M's body their view would compel them to consider it still to have been an open book so far as personhood is concerned. So the Joneses' claim that the baby who emerged from the operating theater was their child despite his outward resemblance to a McDermott, is not supported by the orthodox view.

I do not intend to offer moral judgements about the case of baby J and baby M, either as I have related it or in any other possible way it may have developed. I am concerned neither with the moral propriety of performing operations of the kind I have proposed nor with the moral claims either set of parents might have on the complete baby created by the doctors. Nor am I concerned to comment extensively on the likelihood that a scenario of this kind might ever arise in reality; this is pure fantasy. Or is it? Despite the technical problems that would arise because of the complexity, of the brain, the spinal column and the rest of the nervous system, presumably a minimal possibility exists that brain transplants will one day be possible, though the ethical outrage that might be created by the idea of transplanting living human brains from one body to another might be sufficient to deter anyone from admitting that they had carried out such a procedure. And presumably the ethical outrage that might be caused by the announcement that a chimp's brain had been placed in the skull of an otherwise complete human baby would be even greater. No matter, my intention in creating this scenario and the scenario in which a human baby's body is merged with a chimp baby's brain, has little to do with the world of practical science; and it has little to do with the world of practical ethics.

However, I hope I have demonstrated that the fictitious idea of brain transplants whether between human babies or between human babies and babies of related species, produces some interesting, if unusual, problems when applied to newly born babies. Even more interesting problems might be raised if we were to consider the possibility of carrying out brain transplants on human babies (or fetuses if you would prefer) in the period before birth. Some surgical procedures may already be performed in the ante-natal period and just as we can reflect on the possibility of genetic surgery in which "bad" (or unwanted) genes are swapped for "good," that is, preferred ones, in order to allow us to eradicate genetic conditions that are not valued, I invite you to reflect on the possibility that intra-uterine transplant surgery may one day be possible.

And I invite you to reflect on the perplexing problems that we might face in determining not only who will have "rights" in relation to children who now have been involved in intra-uterine brain transplants (which mirror questions that may be raised at present in relation to babies who are born after both surrogacy and some techniques of reproductive technology) but who such children will be. Will such a child be the child of the mother and father whose procreative endeavors contributed the body or of those who contributed the brain?

NOTES

1. Gavin Fairbairn, "Enforced Life: Enforced Death," *Journal of Medical Ethics* (1991).

2. See, for example, Helga Kushe, *The Sanctity of Life Doctrine in Medicine: A Critique* (Oxford: Oxford University Press, 1987); Helga Kushe and Peter Singer, *Should The Baby Live?* (Oxford: Oxford University Press: 1985); and John Haris, *The Value of Life* (London: Routledge, 1985).

3. Bernard Williams, *Problems of the Self* (Cambridge, England: Cambridge University Press, 1973); Derek Parfit, *Reasons and Persons* (Oxford: Clarendon Press, 1984).

Twelve

DEATH, BRAINS, AND PERSONS

Chris Belshaw

Philosophy is presently much concerned with death. This can only be welcome. A subject which in popular circles has for too long been taboo, and which within professional philosophy has seemed to afford no opportunity for analytic rigor has, in recent years, proved to be of remarkable fecundity in generating and sustaining valuable debate. This is just one manifestation of a general broadening of our concerns, a willingness to tackle again a range of serious and difficult areas. And even if this willingness exists alongside ever narrower specialization elsewhere, this is all to the good: philosophical concerns have never been easily circumscribed, and connections between seemingly remote areas are often unexpectedly fruitful. But although much of this new concern is both promising and healthy, I think this is not true of it all.[1] The focus on the meaning of "death," the interest in fixing the necessary and sufficient conditions under which death can occur, the endeavor to analyze the concepts here involved, has proved, I will argue, to be ill-founded. What we might seek to understand of death has no need of conventional philosophical precision, and is handicapped by the conviction that such precision is appropriate. What we might seek to understand is, I will maintain, fuzzy at the edges. But I will also maintain this gives no cause for alarm.

One way of tackling this issue must be avoided. And that is to meet, head on, the wealth of technical and semi-technical material, both of a philosophical and of a clinical nature, which has been produced over recent years, seeking then to demonstrate, in a necessarily painstaking manner, just where its weaknesses lie, and where its conclusions, even if well argued, fail to engage with matters of genuine philosophical concern.[2] This must be avoided, first, because space does not permit it, but second, because of the serious danger of becoming hopelessly submerged in all this detail. So, while not avoiding altogether some reference to this technical material, the argument is presented in broader strokes, in the hope that its main moral, which is by no means confined to issues of death, surface all the more.

1. A History

Until recently, death has been, in some respects, unproblematic. People became injured or ill, their condition deteriorated abruptly or by degrees, and then, in close succession, consciousness was lost, the heart ceased to beat, blood failed to circulate, organs, the brain critically among them, began to atrophy, and they were correctly pronounced dead. Nor did it much matter if death was diagnosed before all these stages were gone through. After a point, the continuation of such a process is inevitable.

Such was the situation when medicine was in its infancy. And it has for a long time been in essence unchanged. But in recent decades, considerable advances have been made which allow us to interrupt and interfere with this process. Many occasions exist when the heart ceases to beat, but then is encouraged to beat again. Total heart failure need not lead to death, for the heart can be replaced. The heart and lungs can be shut off for long periods, and respiration given over to a machine. Parts of the brain can be removed, leaving the remainder still to function. And the entire brain can cease to function, while, with the aid of machines, the onset of further processes associated with death can be arrested. Technology has a considerable momentum of its own, and it will only be a matter of time before we will be able to intervene in still further ways. Only a matter of time, then, before the entire body can be shut down, and later started again, before transplants of the brain, or parts of the brain, can occur, before we are able to clone a replica of an individual from a mere part. Perhaps not all, but much of what is conceivable will become possible. And even if outcry calls a halt to such experimentation on the human subject, it will continue, and in the end be successful, where other animals are concerned.

Techniques have advanced, and so too has understanding. Mention must be made of our still rudimentary but not altogether unimpressive grasp of the workings of the brain. We know that consciousness, memory, the emotions, reside here, and we know too that the brain regulates the performance of many of the body's other vital organs: the heart, the kidneys, the liver all function under the brain's control. In brief, the brain sustains our life. We know further, something of the disposition of the parts of the brain. I have no need for details: suffice it to say that while the brain stem governs the overall functioning of the brain, and governs too, the proper working of the organism as a whole, the cerebral hemispheres are the seat of consciousness, and thus of the characteristics of the human personality. Damage to the hemispheres can render a human being utterly bereft of the range of mental activity, from reflection on one's past down to the brute sensation of pain, while, so long as the brain stem is operative, the vegetative functions can be sustained.

Knowledge engenders ignorance. In the light of these many advances we now want to ask: When is a person dead? Do those whose hearts fail, but who later recover, in the meantime die, or were they alive throughout? Were we mistaken to think of death as the end? When the heart functions, yet the brain does not, is this death? When the brain stem functions, but the cerebral hemispheres do not, has death occurred?

To many these questions have been of devastating concern. It has seemed critical that we establish precisely what degree of damage to the body's organs, and to the brain, is compatible with life's continuation. For only then can we discover whether those in a coma, or persistent vegetative state, are dead or alive, and only then can we properly decide on the appropriateness of removing organs for use elsewhere, continuing with, or switching off life-support systems, and making, in general terms, best use of scarce resources. And to facilitate our answering such questions it has seemed, in turn, essential that we uncover the precise definition of death. But although such concerns are widespread, they represent, I believe, some considerable confusion. The search for a definition of death is misguided.

I will argue that no substantive philosophical questions arise in this area with which we might engage, no logically necessary and sufficient conditions of death exist to be uncovered, no concept to be usefully analyzed, no metaphysical issue with which to be concerned. But key questions do remain. First, we encounter a range of scientific questions—what exactly happens when respiration fails? How long after the brain is deprived of oxygenated blood does deterioration begin? What is the probability, after such and such damage, of the personality or consciousness, being restored? Second, are the moral questions. For we still want to know whether life should always be sustained, when, if ever, we might remove and reuse bodily organs, or how properly to respond to someone whose vegetative functions persist, while consciousness is gone. Third, are the problems of definition. Under what confluence of clinical conditions ought we to speak of unconsciousness, or coma, or death? What we ought to say depends, in part on what we do say; this definitional issue draws upon a record of everyday practice. A need arises for a kind of anthropology. But philosophy, beyond the worthwhile but unglamorous task of sorting out muddles, and helping bring about, for purely practical reasons, a conceptual tidiness, has here nothing of significance to add. We deceive ourselves and others in claiming otherwise. Or so I will argue.

2. Evidence and Meaning

Does death exist? Assuredly—and in almost every case, the detection of death is straightforward. We do not doubt that Churchill and Kennedy are dead, and conversely, that (as I write) Mandela and Farrakhan are still alive. But the means by which we establish whether a death has occurred depends on the kind of thing being considered. What we look for, in trying to establish whether a person has died, is well-known. We listen to the heart, check for pulse, hold a mirror to the mouth, consider temperature and pallor, and so on. None of this is relevant to a concern for the plants in my garden. Is this wilt? Do I find sap if I cut into their stems? These questions are of little relevance to the fish in the lake. I check to see whether they are swimming, or floating side up on the surface. So what I look for, the evidence with which I am most concerned in trying to establish whether a thing is alive or dead, differs in relation to the sort of creature with which I am concerned. The common signs of death are, then, species-relative.

Does this suggest, as some have supposed, that what we mean by speaking of death itself varies accordingly? Does it suggest that "dead" in "the tadpoles are dead" means something different from (what appears to be) the same word in "Tallis is dead," or "most of our elms are now dead." Surely it does not. What we can say is that the use of different evidential criteria does not itself entail a difference in meaning. No reasons are present, drawn from our use of different evidence, to deny what on the face of it appears to be right: when taken in a literal sense, "is dead" and "death" are univocal. The meaning of death is not species-relative.[3]

Now we are challenged to say just what death means, or what the dead, of any and every species, have in common. Can the challenge be met? I believe it can. "Death" is often taken to mean, I think, something like the "irreversible breakdown of the organism as a whole."

Every term in this account is critical. I will suppose that only organisms can literally die. When we speak of the death of other things, of the author, of God, or the engine of a car, we speak metaphorically. When we speak of the death of a child, or a fern, or a sparrow, we speak literally; we are concerned with the organism as whole. A plant does not die when a flower dies, and nor do I when a tooth dies. Death of a part is not sufficient for death of the whole. Nor is death of every part necessary, for I can surely die while cells, tissues or even entire organs continue to live.

The notion of irreversibility is problematic, but the thinking behind it is intelligible. We shall not normally want to say that a person, or a plant or a parrot is dead, while a chance of recovery is still possible. When death comes, so does despair: we cease our efforts at revival and acquiesce in the present onset of what, in the end, is inevitable for us all. But the issue is hardly resolved. For the notion of chance raises issues of its own. I will return to this below, saying here that we are concerned with what, in some given circumstances, present themselves as genuine possibilities for recovery—the diagnosis of death is not overturned because some logical possibility obtains, or indeed because some physical possibility has, in different but related circumstances, entered into the fray.

What meaning can be attached to "breakdown?" This everyday term should here be understood in its customary sense. So organism breakdown is like automobile breakdown, or a breakdown in transmission just before the evening news—standard operations are not hampered, but are interrupted, and unless the system is sophisticated and self-regulating, intervention is called for before they can be resumed. The car can usually be fixed, finances permitting, and breakdown within human beings is, similarly, often only temporary. Death marks the time when the hiatus becomes permanent.

Death so described is vague. First, a residual unclarity about the kinds of things that can die exists. The boundary between organisms and organic material is, so far, imprecise. Do apples, as opposed to their trees, ever die? Does soil become dead literally, or only metaphorically? Second, even given that we are considering kinds of things which, uncontroversially, do die, unclarity will exist, on occasion, as to whether individuals are dead or alive. Consider human beings. Cases exist (and I describe some in more detail below) with no facts of the matter as to whether our subject is dead or alive. This is not because the facts are themselves somehow imprecise. I believe we can, in principle, describe in full detail the physical condition in which the body finds itself. Further, because we can understand causal relations, we can say, again in principle, what needs to be changed to allow this person again to walk, or to talk, or take tea. We will be able to say whether what needs here to be done can be done, or whether costs, or technology, or physics stands in the way. But from none of this will it follow that the person is dead, or alternatively, alive. If we can describe the physical facts, then we have done all that can be done. Sometimes we cannot adequately describe these facts. We do not know exactly what the body's present condition is, or what will happen if we intervene in such and such ways. But these outstanding questions are clinical. They are not questions with which philosophers can profitably be engaged.

3. Definitions

Consider the following challenge to my account. "You say only organisms can die. Suppose something like Manicheanism is true, and cosmic battle exists between good and evil. And suppose Satan is vanquished. Not only does he retire, temporarily, from the scene. He is utterly destroyed, never to rise again. Evil no longer exists. On your account, we cannot say that Satan is dead. For he is no organism. But how can you insist on saying, we cannot say that?"

I do not need to insist on this. My aim is to indicate how the word is used. Of the types of thing we know to exist, whose existence is temporary, which come and go—and these include rocks and stones, plants, animals, machines, atmospheres, governments, policies, stars—my claim is, we speak of literal death only where organisms are concerned. My account purports to be extensionally correct. It purports to record the ways in which we speak with confidence, noting what we don't, instead of insisting on what we can't say. (We would more readily speak of the vanquishing, the destruction, the non-existence, the conquering of evil, instead of its death). Were it to be different, my account would need revision.

My "definition," then, is in one common sense of the term, no such thing. It does not attempt to provide the logically necessary and sufficient conditions of death, to range over all possible worlds, so gearing us for inter-galactic travel, sorting the living from the dead wherever and whenever we go. Instead, my "definition" is a piecemeal and, I hope, much more modest attempt to capture the shape of our mutterings on this piece of earth as we now find it. So the intention is to describe something of the structure of our practices, instead of to draw limits on where, in future or different circumstances, we might wish to go. To hope for more is vanity.

Room is available for a substantial qualification. It might be thought I am here dismissing the whole, and familiar, apparatus of necessary and sufficient conditions. I do not intend this. Nor do I deny that necessary and sufficient conditions of death exist. But as that may appear to be in flat contradiction of what has just been said, I will explain.

Sufficient conditions are used to identify death. We know that (human) death can be brought about in a variety of ways, by ingesting large amounts of strychnine and no antidote, by being cut into small pieces, and distributed to the winds, or by being left for days, without shelter, at the South Pole. Tell me any such thing has happened to anyone you know, and I will infer with certainty that they are now dead. Necessary conditions are also used: a necessary condition of someone's being dead is that they are not now shopping, discussing politics, reading this, and so on. If your friends are doing any such thing then they are alive.

But first, the examples of sufficient conditions refer to causal, and not logical relations. As a matter of fact, and not logic, we suffer the cold, and are poisoned by some substances, and not by others. Is it similarly a matter of fact that the dead are unable to shop? Or is this now a logical relation? This issue is not straightforward and must, for reasons of space, be set aside. But second, I do not intend that the two sets of conditions can be combined to give us, in the standard sense, necessary and sufficient conditions for someone's being dead. I do not intend, that is, that the coincidence of these conditions might deal with every problem case, either in practice, or in principle. For the necessary conditions mark a broad area beyond which death cannot be found, while the sufficient conditions pick incontrovertible cases within it. Even taken together, a residual area occurs where the question of death is undecided.

Why should anyone think that uncovering definitions, or digging out logically necessary and sufficient conditions for the use of a term is significant? Why does fixing death matter? On a radical view, unless we can do this, we can never say, with warrant, whether someone is dead. This is preposterous. But I fear that among those new to philosophy, it will be too beguiling. On a moderate view, unless we can do this, we cannot always say whether someone is dead. We might come across cases where what we do know, what is well established, is insufficient for determining whether what we now face is dead or alive. This is less preposterous, and, I think, a perfectly acceptable state of affairs—even on the more contentious of the two construals.

On the first, a problem case occurs because of limitations to our knowledge. Is Parkinson's disease caused by a virus? We do not know this yet. But what a virus is, and what the disease consists in, are both well enough known. So, to answer our question, more facts are needed. On the second, no such limitations exist. For our inability to answer a given question, under such a construal, comes about because no answers can be given. We might know all the relevant facts, but from these no resolution of the puzzle will follow. We are often furnished with perfectly adequate information about someone's condition. We can understand to what extent they can feel pain, for example, or how well they react to stimuli. And we can understand how their condition might deteriorate or improve, and know what needs to be done, to prevent such deterioration, or promote such improvement. Again, if gaps exist in our understanding, then we must turn to physicians, neurologists, and the like. In principle, such gaps can be filled. We then find ourselves in a situation where no further medical or clinical information will have a bearing on the case.

We have four options:

(1) Either we think that from these available facts it just follows that a person is dead or alive.

(2) Or we think a further fact exists, of the same order, which is just the fact of their being dead or alive.

(3) Or we think of a further fact, or collection of facts, but of a different order, which are relevant to the situation.

(4) Or, finally, we acknowledge that, in such a case, nothing further can be known, even if, in virtue of this, room is available for a decision, as to how best to describe the case, in light of assorted considerations.

I might make brief comment on each of the options. I claim that, in many cases, it does follow from the intersection of diverse facts that someone is dead, or alive. But no reason arises to make us think that we already have the precision to guarantee this of every case. Nor can I make much sense of the idea that being, say, dead might be a discrete physical fact which obtains or not, independently of other physical facts about the body's condition. The third option represents a favored philosophical stamping ground. For what is often claimed is that although the hunt for garden facts of death is inappropriate, non-standard facts can be found. We confront, that is, a problem in metaphysics. But again, I have immense difficulty in grasping the suggestion that metaphysical facts of death exist to which philosophers, as opposed to scientists, or people in the street have a special access. That leaves the fourth option and, as will become apparent, this is the option I want to endorse.

4. Revival and Time

Our thinking about death labors under difficulties in some areas. One such area, as I noted earlier, concerns the irreversible nature of the process. We will consider this in a little more detail.

Is it possible to revive the dead? Or is death necessarily the end? What we say here has a bearing on our attitude to the resurrection of Christ, and to contemporary freezing and preservation techniques. But although puzzles exist, I want to insist, against some recent philosophers, that no substantive problems arise here.

Again, we can describe the facts well enough. After this, only terminological issues remain. My suspicion, for what it is worth, is that if the ground heaved, the charnel houses opened, and skeletons walked the earth, we would say that the dead have risen. If, in slight contrast, a standard medical procedure were developed for reviving those who today are confidently buried, then we would, over time, cease to think of them as ever having been dead. Thus, supernatural intervention would not, I suspect, make radical alteration to our categorizing, whereas alterations in what is natural, and commonplace, would. An example of this can be seen in the shift in thinking about those whose hearts fail as straightforwardly and immediately dead. A further case, and one discussed in the literature, concerns cryanation. Are the cryanated dead, and awaiting a rebirth? Or has death here been thwarted, even if to no obvious avail? My suspicion, again for it is worth, is that at present we think of these people as dead (and perhaps also as wasteful of their money).[4]

The major point here, however, and the reason that I am not inclined to elaborate further on my suspicions, is that we can in all such cases describe well enough the condition in which these subjects find themselves. We can say, for example, of those who have undergone cryanation, that their organs are in such and such a condition, their body at this or that temperature, and we can, further, describe in some detail exactly what will happen if the machines are turned off, and everything now possible is done to bring about revival. Why should we believe that to do all this is not to do quite enough, and leaves outstanding a further question of whether the subjects are dead or alive? I see no reason to persist in such a belief.

This brings us back to irreversibility. Death is not a condition the reversal of which is logically impossible. No such conditions exist. Is it a condition the reversal of which is physically impossible? Again no. We can possibly revive someone after the heart has stopped. Those whose hearts are so revived are not, at that time, dead. Set aside whether these people are ever dead. Still, we should not say that those whose hearts stopped, some hundred years ago, or whose hearts stop today, but hundreds of miles from a hospital, are not dead. Our current technology does not, I think, reach back into distant times, or over into remote places, overturning decisions made there about who is dead, and who is alive. Our technology is impotent in this respect even though, as what is physically possible does not change, it was possible even then, and is possible even there, for revival to occur. So I maintain someone can be dead, even though it is physically possible for them to live again. Our relation to the past is echoed by the future's relation to us. What is reasonable to suppose is that many conditions which are today irreversible will become reversible with time. Technology will make realizable more and more physical possibilities. But our judgements about who is, and who is not dead, should not be thought of as tentative in virtue of this.

Should we say, then, that death is a condition the reversal of which is technologically impossible? We could then say that those whose hearts failed a century ago were dead, while their counterparts today are alive. And we could say that present decisions about who is dead will not be overturned by future developments. But, inevitably, problems arise. We do not want, I think, to suggest that decisions made in England depend on the state of technology in, say America. And we do not want to say, of those whose bodies are frozen, that they are dead today, but might come back to life in the future, in virtue of technological developments alone. We do not want to say, that is, that they will come back to life even before the new technology is brought to bear upon them.

5. Death, States, and the Brain

Attention to the condition of the brain has, with good reason, been given a greater focus in recent years. Its condition, instead of that of the heart, provides valuable evidence as to whether the subject is dead or alive. And this on numerous counts. First, damage to the brain occurs, in many cases, later than damage to heart, or lungs. Second, brain damage is, in the main, irreversible. Erring on the side of caution is reasonable where the pronouncement of death is concerned. And attention to the brain, given such characteristics, encourages this. But caution might be extreme: the criterion still needs a rationale, which it gets because of the intimate connection between the state of the brain and the bulk of our fundamental concerns. Third, then, what we care about, in caring about human beings, depends on the condition of the brain. Not only can the heart be repaired, it can be, when damage is irreversible, replaced. The brain cannot, in present circumstances, be replaced. But suppose that it could. Mere replacement, even if it would restore a human life, would not preserve the individual whose death represents to us such a loss. Unless we develop also the technology to preserve content then, assuredly, a new brain will leave us with a new personality and so also, under a popular construal, a new person.

These considerations are connected. And what they amount to is this: so long as damage is contained within the heart, a human life might be restored. When damage seriously infects the brain, a human life is, under present conditions, irrevocably lost.

What degree of damage to the brain brings about death? We can speak of the death of the whole brain, and we can speak also of the death of its parts. And this, given the overall structure of the brain, allows for three competing views as to when death comes about. For although a wholly accurate picture is more complex, it can be useful to think of the brain as having two major divisions, consisting of its upper part, comprising in the main the cerebral hemispheres, and a lower part, the brain stem. Now one influential view is that whole brain death is necessary for the death of a human being. The main rival view is that death of the hemispheres alone is sufficient for human death. A further view would be that death of the brain stem alone is sufficient for death. This view is of theoretical interest only. For, in practice, no cases are encountered where the brain stem is dead, while the upper brain lives on. However, many inverse cases exist, where the upper brain dies, but the stem remains alive. Such is the situation befalling those people in a persistent vegetative state; those who (so far as we can tell) will never again regain consciousness, and in whom the unconscious life is equally stultified, but whose other organs will, with some assistance by way of feeding and care, continue to function in a regular and coherent fashion. Reflection on the pity of such a condition, and the problem of how best to cope with it, stands behind much of our recent concern with understanding death.

Where, in all this, is a criterion of death to be found? Those who argue that whole brain death is logically necessary and sufficient for human death make a gross mistake. That our heads are full of glass is a logical possibility. Conversely, living brains, or brain parts, might happily exist in complete isolation from the remainder of the human being, functioning, in their happy isolation, as tomatoes do now. So we set logic aside. Those who argue that we are here considering a causal relationship make a mistake, but of a lesser kind. The physical possibility exists to keep parts of the brain alive under laboratory conditions for a designated period. Moral scruples intervene where human subjects are concerned, but many such experiments use animals. No one would think that if a rat's brainstem is alive in a jar, then so too is the rat. Nor would anyone have the corresponding thought about a human being. Whole brain death cannot be physically necessary for death of the individual. Can it be sufficient?

Consider what is for now a hypothetical case. Perhaps it may be physically possible to remove and dispose of the whole brain from patient A, and replace it with the brain from patient B, then for A to walk and talk again. A's brain is dead. Whether A is dead is unclear, even if it is apparent that, unless we are able to attend to content, A's previous character, beliefs and memories, no longer exist. We might want to say, then, that someone can survive the death of their brain.

This is, however, a lesser mistake, for though we rule out the possible occurrence of arcane circumstances, it remains the case that whole brain death remains a viable criterion, and a more accurate measure in practice, than earlier heart-lung criteria, of when death occurs. We can say with full confidence that when the whole brain is dead, so too is the human being. But granted that we have what is for practical purposes a sufficient condition, the question that remains is whether whole brain death provides also a (practically) necessary condition of death of the human being. This has been proposed, but might it be too cautious? Might we not have ample reason to hold that the human being is dead, even while life in the lower brain continues? Might not death of the upper brain be not only (practically) necessary for death of the human being, but itself sufficient?

I want here to side with the conservatives. While allowing a theoretical possibility of sustaining just the brain stem, while all life elsewhere is gone, the practical issue we are faced with is different. For the practical issue is precisely that described above, in the account of someone in a persistent vegetative state. Survival of the lower brain occurs not in isolation, but is usually connected with survival of a nexus of human vegetative functions. To me, the most appropriate way of describing this is to say the human being continues to live, but, because of damage to the upper brain, is now and hereafter, in a parlous condition. Those in a persistent vegetative state are, then, not dead.

Here a distinction is introduced which will strike some immediately as sophistical. For some will now want to distinguish between the person and the human being, insisting that even if the human being lives on, the person has, in such a circumstance, died.[5] The problems with such a proposal are well known—it requires that we have two discrete entities, which occupy the same space, and whose lives are for the most part intimately connected, but one of which may predecease the other. But some degree of sympathy with the proposal is appropriate. The alteration brought to a human being by substantial damage to the upper brain is immense, causing total and permanent loss of consciousness and personality. We might, with reason, here speak of the person's no longer existing, even while the human being remains alive. But to speak of the death of the person is still under-motivated. We are inclined, as I have said, to speak of death in connection with biological entities, and while we may ordinarily think of persons as entities of this kind, we should no longer persist in that once a person/human being distinction is introduced. But suppose we do persist. Non-biological entities can cease to exist without dying, and some biological entities can also do this. Such is the everyday fate of acorns, amoebae, caterpillars, and the like. And such is our fate in a host of science fiction films. So even were we to maintain both that the person no longer exists, and that persons are biological entities, still no need would exist to insist that the person had died.

The introduction of a distinction between persons and human beings helps, I think, to take further an issue left hanging above. Suppose A's body does get B's brain, with no adjustment to content. I said that it remains unclear whether A is dead or alive. One view is A continues to live, but is much changed. Another is A no longer exists, even if the body still does. And some thinkers, connecting life of an individual with the life of a brain, will want to say that in this case A is dead, while others, appealing to the distinction, will insist only that the person A is gone, while the human being lives on. What is the truth here?

My major point is that we err in thinking a truth exists. We can describe all the facts. We can say what the body is like, where the two brains now are, how well the parts fit together, what traits, seeming-memories and beliefs, survive the operation, and so on. Once we have done this, the question of whether A is dead, or has by some other means gone out of existence, is verbal. We can say what we like. Attempts might be made to breathe life into what is seen as a real issue here by asking whether the evil scientist who deals with A in such a way will be charged with murder. But this is futile. What has happened to A is, so far as he is concerned, as bad as death. What the scientist does is as bad as murder. Further than this we cannot go. We can equally say what we like in the real situations with which we are already concerned. I think those in a persistent vegetative state are alive. But I will not attempt to prove this. Once the facts are agreed on, room is available for a decision as to how best to speak on the matter of life or death. A proof that we should go one way or the other is not something we can hope to attain.

6. Persons and Morals

I said at the outset that the moral I want to draw is general. Some hint of that has already been made in referring, as I did above, to the analogous problems with the definition of art. Now I might mention, though briefly, a further area where, or so I claim, we look in vain for physical or metaphysical truth, argue at length about the matter, and persist in thinking that when and only when such truths are uncovered, answers to further of our questions will be resolved. I have needed in the previous discussion to make reference to persons; and I have proceeded, in the main, as though persons form a category of their own, non-biological perhaps, but whose members might with considerable precision be identified, described, and distinguished from near-cousins and impostors alike. I have no need to retract any of this, but possibly some of it might lead to misinterpretations.

Do persons exist? Assuredly—you are one, and I am an other. Just as assuredly, things which are not persons exist—for a range of examples, any of the objects on my desk. But does a definition of personhood exist, a means of picking out persons in all possible worlds, or even more modestly, hard and fast criteria for their foolproof identification in this world? I think not. Though we can properly speak of persons in a range of circumstances, a fact of the matter as to whether what we consider a person or non-person is not in every case. But again, we can describe in ample detail just what it is we do consider, discuss, with appropriate precision, just where it has been, and where it is going, and characterize, with sufficient clarity, exactly what it is, and what it is not, capable of doing, or thinking, or feeling. Thereafter, no questions of substance need be addressed.

So the abortion question does not, contrary to widespread opinion, rest on the issue of whether the fetus is a person. The opposing factions are involved in a pseudo-debate, falsely believing they engage in some scientific or metaphysical dispute, when the only issue is how best to classify these entities which fall, in altogether accountable ways, between evident non-persons, and incontrovertible persons.[6] Similarly, for the debate about those suffering from severe forms of dementia. Both the question of whether we have here some person or other, and the question of whether any such person is to be identified with the person we previously knew are illusory. We can say well enough what this human being is able now to do, how much of their character and memory. connects with that previously displayed. In this case, we have done all we can, leaving only some classification problems, the resolution of which is of minor importance.

But why, if these questions of death and personhood are so obvious, have they been so long and so vigorously debated? Remember, I said that some types of questions do survive. Among these are moral questions. My deep suspicion is, first, that the answer to these moral questions is not determined by reference to any set of factual questions and second, that this is an uncomfortable truth that we are less than willing to face.

Consider, then, the question of organ removal. Were it permissible to remove organs only from the dead, then the question of whether those in a persistent vegetative life are dead or alive would be of critical importance. Given such a moral precept, we would well understand the motivation of those who argue that such people are dead already. For, seeking to make use of the organs, little option would exist but to argue that their hosts are no longer of this world. Similarly, if the killing of innocent persons is always wrong, then to demonstrate the fetus's personhood will secure the conservative position on abortion against that of their rivals.

If our moral precepts have, then, this tidy form, and moral distinctions are to be imposed where, within the world, some factual distinction obtains, we will need to settle these factual matters. But, I have argued, where the facts are concerned clarity is ambiguous. Neither as a matter of science nor of metaphysics can we draw an exact line between the living and the dead. Nor does such a line exist between persons and non-persons; nor, though I have not discussed this here, between human beings and members of other species. This throws the moral and value questions into stark relief. So, instead of making a commitment to such moral injunctions, and thereafter supposing that factual matters are the ones at issue we should, I recommend, acknowledge that ethical dilemmas are those we must face.

What has to be decided, is, might we remove the organs of someone who has lost all hope of a worthwhile life, someone who will never talk, think, or feel pain again, but whose heart, and lungs and kidneys might, with some assistance, continue to function? We cannot avoid this by considering, instead, whether the person is dead or alive. The moral questions do not track, as easily as we might hope, these life and death issues. Similarly for abortion. Is termination wrong? That question is not to be decided by discovering whether the fetus is a person. Nothing of that kind can be discovered. Once we realize how messy and how *sui generis* is the network of facts which here obtain—no self consciousness, a degree of sentience, but immense potential—then the moral dilemma, with all of its difficulties, is more accurately grasped.

The moral questions, so understood, might appear intractable. We have room for optimism so long as answers to some factual questions are outstanding. For we might think once they are settled agreement will be mandatory. If the fetus were a person, some liberals allow, abortion would be wrong. But it is not. Similarly, some conservatives agree that if those in a persistent vegetative state were dead, organ removal would be permissible. But they are not. Hanging the issues on factual questions sustains hope of consensus somewhere down the line. For we can think that once the facts are established all reasonable people must surely agree on what is to be done. What we need to see, however, or so I have argued, is that we can establish, and agree on all relevant factual matters, and yet leave the moral issues unresolved. How then to resolve them? That is the difficulty we must be prepared to face.

NOTES

1. See the papers in J. M. Fischer, *The Metaphysics of Death* (Stanford: Stanford University Press, 1993), and also those collected in *The Monist*, 76:2 (1993).

2. See Karen Gervais, *Redefining Death* (New Haven: Yale University Press, 1986); David Lamb, *Death, Brain Death, and Ethics* (London: Routledge, 1985); Michael B. Green and Daniel Wikler, "Brain Death and Personal Identity," *Philosophy and Public Affairs*, 9 (1981); President's Commission for the Study of Ethical Problems in Medicine and Biomedical and Behavioral Research, *Defining Death* (Washington: U.S. Government Printing Office, 1981).

3. See Fred Feldman, *Confrontations with the Reaper* (Oxford: Oxford University Press, 1992).

4. *Ibid.*

5. See John Lizza, "Persons and Death: What's Metaphysically Wrong with Our Current Statutory Definition of Death?", *Journal of Medicine and Philosophy*, 18 (1993).

6. See Richard Dworkin, *Life's Dominion: An Argument about Abortion and Euthanasia* (London: Harper Collins, 1993).

Thirteen

DEFINING DEATH: A BIOLOGICAL OR CULTURAL MATTER?

John P. Lizza

The "personhood argument" for the higher-brain formulation of death holds that the capability for cognitive function is a necessary condition of personhood, and that death occurs when a person loses this faculty.[1] Advocates of the personhood argument view cognitive function as dependent on or identical to some higher-brain functions, and when those brain functions cease, the person dies. Under the higher-brain formulation, individuals in persistent vegetative state (PVS), who have irreversibly lost all higher-brain functions but have retained functions of the brain stem such as the regulation of breathing and heartbeat, should therefore be considered dead. A breathing human body is not itself a person, and without a functioning neocortex, individuals in PVS are just breathing bodies.

Some bioethicists reject the higher-brain formulation of death because they claim it violates a requirement that "death" should mean the same thing when applied to human beings as when applied to other species.[2] The influential President's Commission for the Study of Ethical Problems in Medicine and Biomedical and Behavioral Research agreed with this claim and argued further that the whole-brain formulation of death, as opposed to the higher-brain formulation, was consistent with the traditional, purely biological, trans-species concept of death.[3] Fred Feldman has also recently claimed that "death" is a biological concept and univocal for all living organisms.[4] Feldman asks us to consider the following three sentences:

(1) JFK died in November 1963.

(2) The last dodo bird died in April 1681.

(3) My oldest Baldwin apple tree died during the winter of 1986.

No reason exists to suppose that the word "died" has one meaning in sentence (1) and different meanings in the other two sentences. No special meaning of death is applicable to persons or other higher-order organisms, which the higher-brain formulation of death requires.

In this chapter, I challenge the assumption that the concept of death is purely biological and univocal for all living organisms. I do so by first looking at the rationale behind the President's Commission's acceptance of the whole-brain criterion of death and the definition of death accepted by the Commission. I next argue that consideration of the locked-in syndrome shows that the definition of death accepted by the Commission fails. I then consider two alternative, biological definitions of death that have been proposed respectively by Lawrence Becker and Jay Rosenberg.[5] I argue that consideration of PVS and the hypothetical case of an artificially sustained, decapitated human body shows that their biological definitions also fail. I further argue that any definition of death for human beings or persons is tied to conceptions of humanity and personhood that go beyond biological taxonomy and biological definitions of life and death. Finally, building on what I find sensible in Rosenberg's account, I propose a definition of death that is explicitly linked to conceptions of humanity and personhood.

In short, because of technological interventions in the life-history of human beings and persons, "death" can no longer be viewed as a univocal, purely biological concept. Human beings and persons can now die in ways that previously were impossible. These new ways of dying are made possible by medical technology. What it means to die is relative to the kind of thing that is alive, and to the kind of medical intervention that may be present. Technology has enabled biological entities to live in ways that previously were impossible. They can also, therefore, die in ways that were previously impossible.

Although the President's Commission endorsed a brain-based criterion of death in addition to the traditional heart and lung criterion, the Commission claimed that the brain-based criterion does not introduce a new concept of death, but provides another means for determining when death, as traditionally understood, occurs. The rationale the Commission offered was that it viewed death in the traditional sense as meaning the loss of integration of the organism as a whole. Just as the permanent loss of heart and lung functions marks the loss of integration of the organism as a whole, so, the Commission argued, the loss of all brain function marks the loss of organic integration. Death occurs when functions essential to the maintenance of the organism as an organism, as opposed to a collection of organic parts, permanently cease. James Bernat, Charles Culver, and Bernard Gert later formulated this idea in terms of the following formal definition of death: "the permanent cessation of the functioning of the organism (a living biological entity) as a whole."[6] Bernat, Culver, and Gert, later joined by Alexander Capron and Joanne Lynn, argue that this definition captures what death means for any type of organism.

Stuart Younger and Edward Bartlett, however, point out that the rationale behind this definition of death does not support the whole-brain criterion of death that the Commission, Bernat, and others endorse.[7] Instead, it only supports adoption of a more limited brainstem criterion, since it is the brainstem, not neocortical structures, that are responsible for integrating the organism in a life-sustaining way. In addition, because "the permanent cessation of the functioning of the organism as a whole" is supposed to capture the idea that any organism dies when it loses its internal, organic integration, what is unclear is why it should be thought necessary that higher-brain-functions must cease, since those functions are not essential to the integration of the organism as a whole. Higher-brain-functions would appear to be as necessary to the functioning of the organism as a whole, like fingernail growth. Precisely because the proponents of the above definition do not regard higher-brain functions as necessary for the integration of the organism as a whole, they do not regard individuals in PVS as dead.

The point is that the trans-species definition of death accepted by the Commission, Bernat, and others entails that higher-brain functions are unnecessary to the continued existence of the human organism as a whole, and therefore the loss of integrative organic functions (the breakdown of the heart-lung-brainstem system) suffices for death. The problem with this definition, however, as Younger and Bartlett have pointed out, is that it has the absurd implication that patients with locked-in syndrome are dead. In the locked-in syndrome, the portions of the brain responsible for consciousness and cognition are intact, but those portions of the brain responsible for integration of vegetative functions have been destroyed. The patient with locked-in syndrome has died in the trans-species sense of "the permanent cessation of the organism as a whole," even though this patient retains cognitive function through the efforts of the Intensive Care Unit.

If we think that the patient with locked-in syndrome has not died, then we need to amend the proposed definition of trans-species organic death. If the locked-in patient is still alive, even though the brainstem no longer functions spontaneously and its functions are sustained by mechanical intervention, then whether the brainstem functions are spontaneous in the determination of death is irrelevant. If the human organism has not died in cases of locked-in syndrome (perhaps because we think that persons can not be sustained by dead bodies or because of spontaneous heartbeat and organic functions), then spontaneous brainstem function is unnecessary for human organic life to continue. This is what many who reject any brain-based criterion of death have argued.

Lawrence Becker, for example, holds that "a human organism is dead when, for whatever reason, the system of those reciprocally dependent processes which assimilate oxygen, metabolize food, eliminate wastes and keep the organism in relative homeostasis are arrested in a way which the organism ... cannot reverse."[8] Karen Gervais rightly observes that:

> Becker's definition of organic death refers to the integrated function of the human body; if such functioning persists, whether spontaneously or mechanically assisted, the human being is still alive. The iron lung patient

> is still alive for the same reason that the totally brain dead, respirator driven body is alive: 'the system of...reciprocally dependent processes remains functional.'[9]

Others have also invoked a kind of common sense intuition about death that they claim underlies the traditional heart and lung criterion of death and rejects any brain-based criterion. Paul Quay, for example, asks us to consider two conditions of a woman whose brain has irreversibly ceased to function but who has been placed on a ventilator and other life support.

> Condition 1: (The woman) ... is profoundly unresponsive to any stimulus of pain or pleasure and is quite unable to breathe (i.e., move rib-cage or diaphragm) without the ventilator. But this patient's heart is beating. Her respiration (i.e., exchange of oxygen for gaseous wastes in the lungs and body tissues) continues. Her color is normal brown or pink. Her temperature holds its own against room-temperature, and she sweats if the room is too warm. Her kidneys continue to put out urine. Her leg will kick if the knee is tapped. More strikingly, if she is pregnant, the child continues to grow healthily in her womb. Her body, to be brief, continues to function as one single organism, though none of its functions show any influence of sensation or thought, for which the brain's activity would be needed.
>
> Condition 2: After a few hours or days, a week at longest if we are speaking of an adult, even though the ventilator and the rest of the life-support system continue their activity, the heart stops; the vascular system collapses; respiration halts; the color turns bluish or gray; body-temperature approaches room-temperature; kidneys and other organs cease to function; all reflex movements disappear; the child in the womb will die if not delivered at once by Caesarian section. In a short time, rigor mortis sets in, followed by all the other usual signs of death.[10]

Quay submits that Condition 2 "is the condition people have always designated as 'death.' Condition 1 has hitherto been considered the condition of a living person who is dying of some mortal injury to the brain." Because Conditions 1 and 2 are medically, physiologically, and biologically completely different, Quay sees no reason to label them by the same name, "death." Only Condition 2 can correctly be labelled "death."

In sum, Becker's biological definition of death avoids the unacceptable implication entailed by the definition of Bernat and others: that the locked-in patient has died. It also meets the desideratum that human death means the same thing as the death of any other biological organism. It also recognizes that significant medical, physiological, and biological differences exist between

Quay's Conditions 1 and 2, and supports the common sense view that only individuals in Condition 2 are dead.

Gervais, however, has pointed out that Becker's definition faces two major difficulties.[11] The first is a dilemma: either Becker's proposal is logically inconsistent or it entails the unacceptable idea that death is a reversible process. Gervais argues that when respiratory or cardiac devices are used to restore the integrative functioning of the human body, what is unclear is that those functions have not been "arrested in a way which the organism...cannot reverse." However, if we say that the functions have been arrested in a way in which the organism cannot reverse, then we must say that the organism has died. But then if we intervene mechanically to restore integrative functioning, we will have brought the dead back to life. Contrary to what Gervais holds to be the common assumption that death is irreversible, on Becker's view, death becomes a reversible process. Gervais is unwilling to accept this idea.

The second difficulty for Becker's view, according to Gervais:

> is best demonstrated with a hypothetical case. Becker's position commits us to the claim that someone who has been decapitated, yet whose body is being maintained so that those reciprocally dependent processes which assimilate oxygen, metabolize food, eliminate wastes, and keep the organism in relative homeostasis continue in stride, is alive. Surely we cannot abide this conclusion. A view such as Becker's overlooking as it does the maintenance of organic life, commits him to this absurd consequence.[12]

Gervais's objections are strong, but not because these consequences are as absurd as Gervais thinks. Becker could respond by asking: What is wrong with thinking that a decapitated body sustained by artificial means is a living organism? We would not have a dead body in Quay's condition 2. Becker could also maintain that we should give up the idea that death is irreversible. Perhaps current technology does enable us to bring the organically dead back to life, and the common assumption that death is irreversible is mistaken.

However, even if we suppose that an artificially sustained, decapitated human body would be alive in Becker and Quay's biological sense, whether we would recognize that biological entity to be a human being or human organism is unclear. Indeed, we would not. If decapitation is not enough, consider removing the limbs, so that all that remained was a torso. If that is not enough, consider the artificial maintenance of a system of only those human organs necessary to assimilate oxygen, metabolize food, and eliminate wastes. Technology would have created, in a sense, a new kind of entity—one that fails to satisfy our concept of a human being as a natural kind.[13]

Difficulties emerge in characterizing what metaphysically would be going on if we artificially sustained a decapitated human body, and held that such a living body was not a human being, but some other kind of being. Let us call this new kind of entity a "humanoid." It has human characteristics, but falls short of being human. What type of change did the human being undergo? Did the human being die? Or should we say that the humanoid has lost some abilities and qualities which earlier made it a human being?

At this point, we need to recall why Bernat, Culver, and Gert reject the higher-brain formulation of death and therewith the idea that a person has "died" in PVS.[14] According to them, such an assertion involves a category mistake: a failure to distinguish between (1) an organism ceasing to be a person and (2) an organism dying. Culver and Gert write:

> The alternative definition (that is, the higher-brain definition of death) actually states what it means for that person to die. *Person* is not a biological concept but rather a concept defined in terms of certain kinds of abilities and qualities of awareness. It is inherently vague. Death is a biological concept. Thus, in a literal sense, death can be applied directly only to biological organisms and not to persons. We do not object to the phrase 'death of a person,' but the phrase in common usage actually means the death of the organism which was the person.... By our analysis, Veatch (1975) and others have used the phrase 'death of a person' metaphorically, applying it to an organism which has ceased to be a person but has not died.[15]

Perhaps, paraphrasing the way Bernat, Culver, and Gert characterize the change that occurs when a human being loses personhood in PVS, we should adopt a similar strategy in the case of the artificially sustained, decapitated human body. Perhaps we should distinguish between (1) an organism (the humanoid) ceasing to be a human and (2) an organism dying. The humanoid has not died in Becker and Quay's sense; it has just lost some abilities and qualities necessary to be a human being. Perhaps we should borrow further from Culver and Gert and say the following:

> Human is not a biological concept but rather a concept defined in terms of certain kinds of abilities and qualities. It is inherently vague. Death is a biological concept. Thus, in a literal sense, death can be applied directly only to biological organisms and not to humans. We do not object to the phrase 'death of a human being,' but the phrase in common usage actually means the death of the organism which was the human.... To say that 'a human being has died' is to use the phrase 'death of a human being' metaphorically, applying it to an organism which has ceased to be a human being but has not died.[16]

The point of these remarks is not to argue that we would adopt this strategy, if faced with an artificially sustained, decapitated human body. Instead, it shows that such a strategy is mistaken. If in this case there is a mistake, then such mistakes also arise in analogous treatments of the change that a person undergoes when it sustains PVS.

In the case of an artificially sustained decapitated human body, we would say that the human being has died, and there would be nothing metaphorical about saying so. We would also insist that human being is a biological concept, and not defined in terms of functions or some abilities and qualities of life. We would also have to admit that our concept possesses some vagueness, since it would be hard to draw a sharp distinction between a human being and a humanoid.

The analogy that humanoid is to human what human being is to person shows what is wrong with Bernat and other's dismissal of the higher-brain formulation of death. Bernat and others are no more justified in their claim that proponents of the higher-brain formulation fail to appreciate the significance of the distinction between an organism ceasing to be a person and that organism dying, than we would be justified in claiming that Bernat and others fail to appreciate the distinction (evident in the artificially sustained, decapitated human body) between an organism ceasing to be a human being and that organism dying. If Bernat and others are to hold that person is not a biological concept and that death applies only to biological organisms, then they must admit that human being is not a biological concept, and that therefore "death" cannot be applied to human beings. To avoid this difficulty, they would have to show that human being is not as vague a concept as person, or that we should consider the artificially sustained, decapitated human body to be a human being and not a humanoid.

Both alternatives are implausible. Since persons and human beings are social-historical beings, the biology of persons and human beings is not reducible to animal biology, but is, what Marx Wartofsky has called, "funny biology."[17] Wartofsky's point is that the death of persons and human beings, unlike the death of other types of organisms, is "a socially constituted fact requiring a judgment." The lines drawn between persons, humans, and humanoids, as well as the boundaries of the life and death of these biological entities, are determined by biological considerations and cultural convention. Because these concepts are in part culturally determined, they have a "vagueness" about them that is not found in pure biological taxonomy and biological definitions of life and death.

Consistent with the idea that cultural judgment is involved in fixing the boundaries of our concepts of person, human, and humanoid, what is highly implausible is that our culture would support the judgment that an artificially sustained, decapitated human body was a human being. Even orthodox Jewish law, one of the more conservative positions in the debate over the definition of death, recognizes decapitation as death.[18]

In sum, consideration of the artificially sustained decapitated human being, the locked-in patient, and PVS support the idea that death cannot be defined in the strictly biological terms of the Presidential Commission, Culver, and Gert, or Becker.

I would like to now consider Jay Rosenberg's view that death is a change in kind—the living person changes into a corpse, and that death is the loss of autonomous, global syntropic ability that is permanent and irreversible.[19] I wish to retain Rosenberg's idea that death is a change in kind, but suggest that other ways can be found in which a person can undergo a change in kind without being changed into a corpse, and that these other changes in kind constitute the death of the person. I will also suggest that what it means for an entity to lose its "autonomous, global syntropic ability" is relative to the nature of that entity.

By "syntropic ability" Rosenberg means "the ability of a living organism to preserve or even increase its structural organization through causal transactions with its environment." Although at times he suggests that this syntropic ability or condition of life must be "autonomous" and located in the organism "left to its own devices," he does not consider individuals whose lives are dependent on pacemakers, iron lungs, or kidney dialysis, and who therefore lack independent "syntropic ability," as dead. What is unclear to me is what he would say about some of the cases I have presented in this paper: PVS, "post-mortem" pregnancy, and the artificially sustained, decapitated human body. Seemingly each of these organisms retains syntropic ability, though not independent syntropic ability, and therefore should not be considered "dead" on his view. Each of these organisms do not decay and break down through interaction with the environment in the way a corpse does. The changes that these entities undergo are not the same as the change from a living person to a corpse.

The changes that these organisms undergo are either changes in kind or changes in quality. If they are changes in quality, then, assuming with Rosenberg that death is a change in kind, death has not occurred. As noted earlier, this is the tack that Culver and Gert take in rejecting the higher brain formulation of death. For them, "person" refers to some abilities and qualities of awareness that a human organism might have. In PVS, the human organism has lost those abilities and qualities of awareness, and therefore has ceased to be a person. However, no substantial change in kind has taken place, and death has not occurred. An example would be similar to a person losing the ability to play basketball. We could say that the basketball player no longer exists, but not that a death has occurred.

I argued, however, that a similar tack could be taken in the case in which we artificially sustain a decapitated body. We could construe a human being as a qualitative specification of some other underlying sort, say, humanoid, and argue that a death has not occurred in this case of decapitation. Intuitions about whether a death has occurred in this case, however, run counter to this interpretation. Most of us would say that a death has occurred. So, unless these intuitions are mistaken or unless we have some reason for thinking that PVS is a qualitative change, whereas decapitation is a change in kind, we should be suspicious of the claim that PVS is a qualitative change in the organism, and that death has not occurred.

Alternatively, the changes resulting from PVS, loss of all brain functions, or decapitation may be changes in kind. We then need to ask whether a change in kind entails that a death has occurred.

Rosenberg denies this entailment. He allows for the possibility that an organism can undergo a change in number or kind without dying. He cites examples of an amoeba splitting (a change in number) and of a caterpillar changing into a butterfly (a change in kind). Through these types of changes, he claims, "no life is lost." In contrast, life is not conserved through the change of kind which is death. Perhaps, we should construe the changes resulting from persistent vegetative state, loss of all brain function, and decapitation as changes in which life is conserved and in which death does not occur. Therefore, as in the above examples, a person's life might end when the person irreversibly loses higher brain functions or all brain functions, or is decapitated, but that does not entail that a death has occurred, and that life has not persisted through these types of change.

However, two problems exist with this line of thought. First, Rosenberg's single example of a change in kind of organism without death (the metamorphosis of a caterpillar into a butterfly) is problematic, since the caterpillar is the larva of a butterfly—the earliest stage in the growth of a butterfly, and the metamorphosis is a change in the structure and habits of the insect during normal growth. No change in kind takes place. Instead there has been a change in phase of development. Caterpillar and butterfly are phase sorts of the kind Lepitoptera, instead of different substantial sorts. We are left with the question of whether a change in kind of a living organism can occur without a death occurring.

Second, problems arise in saying that life is conserved through these types of changes that a person might undergo. To say that life *simpliciter* is conserved is not helpful, since one could maintain that life is conserved even through the change of a person into a corpse. Cells in our body still continue to function even after death. Some syntropic ability at the cellular level remains. Some life is conserved even through the change of a person into a corpse.

What we need to do, therefore, is specify the kind of life that is conserved through the change. The syntropic ability of a living person or human organism is presumably not conserved through its change into a corpse. However, if we must specify the kind of life that is not conserved through death, then what is not apparent is that we should say that the life of a person is conserved through loss of higher-brain-functions, and that a death has not occurred with this type of change. The syntropic abilities necessary for the life of a person are different from those of other organisms, and what it means for a person to retain its systemic integrity is different from what it means for other types of organisms to retain their systemic integrity. The activity necessary for the life of a person would include minimally some cognitive ability.

The same point could be made with respect to the change that an organism undergoes when it sustains loss of all brain functions, but is maintained on artificial "life" support, for example, Quay's case of maternal brain death or post-mortem pregnancy. Should we construe the loss of all brain functions as a change in kind in which the life of the human organism is conserved, or should we construe it as a change in kind that is equivalent to death? The pregnant, human organism retains syntropic ability, so much so that it can sustain the life of another organism—the fetus, but to have lost the syntropic ability that we normally associate with a human being. The artificially supported body cannot sustain and increase its structural organization in ways that normal human beings can. So, we should say that a death has occurred, and that another kind of entity—an artifactual entity—is being sustained.

The same argument could be made in the case of an artificially sustained, decapitated human being. Instead of understanding this as a change in kind that does not entail death and in which human life is preserved, we should view it as a substantial change in kind equivalent to the death of the human being, and as the maintenance of some other kind of living entity.

It may be helpful to also make this same point in the context of a critique of Culver and Gert's definition of death as the loss of integration of the organism as a whole. What we mean by "as a whole" is up for grabs. Many thinkers would argue that a person ceases to function "as a whole" when they irreversibly lose all cognitive function, and therefore, *contra* Culver and Gert, the death of a person occurs when there has been an irreversible loss of all cognitive function even though other biological, integrative functions remain. What it means for a person or human being to function "as a whole" would seem to be tied to views about personhood and humanity, and not something that can be settled on purely biological grounds.

The upshot of this analysis is that it requires us to specify the kind of life that lives and dies, and that once we do this, we see that what constitutes the life and death of a person or a human being is tied to conceptions of personhood and humanity that go beyond biological taxonomy and biological definitions of life and death. Death can be defined as a change in kind of living entity marked by the loss of some essential property. The criteria for the death of a person or human being will therefore be determined by the loss of whatever properties are deemed essential to the nature of persons or human beings. In addition, what is deemed essential to the nature of a person or human being will vary with different metaphysical, religious, or other cultural beliefs.

Finally while variations exist in cultural beliefs regarding the nature of a person or human being, there is a remarkable consistency in the Western philosophical tradition in support of the idea that some cognitive function is essential for personhood. While philosophers in the Western tradition have defined persons differently and have suggested different properties as essential to personhood, general agreement exists that some cognitive function is a necessary condition for being a person. For example, Aristotle claimed that persons are rational and social animals; Descartes, that thinking is essential to the nature of a person; Locke, that a person is an object aware of its progress and persistence through time; Hume, that persons are bundles of psychological characteristics; Kant, that persons are rational agents who, among other things, can synthesize experience and act on moral principles; and Sartre, that persons are self-conscious, intentional beings. What all these philosophers have in common is the belief that some type of cognitive function is necessary for something to be a person. Any being devoid of the potential for cognitive function would by implication lack each of the characteristics that these philosophers use to define persons.

Since the neurophysiological basis of any of the cognitive functions that typical persons manifest is destroyed in the case of individuals in PVS, an implied consensus has arisen among philosophers in the Western tradition that they are not persons.[20] Finally, if death is a change in kind of living entity marked by the loss of an essential property, then the philosophical tradition strongly supports the claim that a person who has irreversibly lost all cognitive function has died.

NOTES

1. John Lizza, "Persons and Death: What's Metaphysically Wrong with Our Current Statutory Definition of Death?", *Journal of Medicine and Philosophy,* 18 (1993); H. T. Engelhardt, Jr., "Defining Death: A Philosophical Problem for Medicine and Law," *American Review of Respiratory Diseases*, 112 (1975); Michael Green and Daniel Wikler, "Brain Death and Personal Identity," *Philosophy and Public Affairs*, 9 (1980).

2. See James L. Bernat, Charles M. Culver, and Bernard Gert, "Defining Death in Theory and Practice," *Hastings Center Report*, 12:1 (1982); Alexander Capron and Joanne Lynn, "Reply to J. Smith's Letter to the Editor," *Hastings Center Report*, 12 (1982); James Downie, "Brain Death and Brain Life: Rethinking the Connection," *Bioethics*, 4 (1990); David Lamb, *Death, Brain Death, and Ethics* (Albany, N.Y.: State University of New York Press, 1985).

3. President's Commission for the Study of Ethical Problems in Medicine and Biomedical and Behavioral Research. *Defining Death* (Washington: U. S. Government Printing Office, 1981).

4. Fred Feldman, *Confrontations with the Reaper* (New York: Oxford University Press, 1992).

5. Lawrence C. Becker, "Human Being: The Boundaries of the Concept," *Philosophy and Public Affairs*, 4:4 (1975); and Jay F. Rosenberg, *Thinking Clearly About Death* (Englewood Cliffs, N.J.: Prentice-Hall, 1983).

6. Bernat, Culver, and Gert, "Defining Death in Theory and Practice,"; see also their "Reply to Robert Veatch's Letter to the Editor," *Hastings Center Report*, 12:6 (1982).

7. Stuart Younger and Edward Bartlett, "Human Death and High Technology: The Failure of the Whole-Brain Formulations," *Annals of Internal Medicine*, 99 (1983).

8. Becker, "Human Being," p. 353.

9. Karen Gervais, *Redefining Death* (New Haven: Yale University Press, 1986), p. 54.

10. Paul M. Quay, S.J., "The Hazards of 'Brain-Death' Statutes," *Ethics and Medics*, 18:6 (1993).

11. Gervais, *Redefining Death*, ch. 3.

12. *Ibid.*, p. 57.

13. Hilary Putnam, "Is Semantics Possible?" in *Languages, Beliefs, and Metaphysics*, ed. K. Kiefer and M. Munitz (Albany, N.Y.: State University of New York Press, 1970); Saul Kripke, "Naming and Necessity," in *Semantics of Natural Languages*, ed. Donald Davidson and Gilbert Harman (Dordrecht: Reidel, 1972); and David Wiggins, *Sameness and Substance* (Cambridge, Mass.: Harvard University Press, 1980).

14. Bernat, Culver, and Gert, "Reply to Robert Veatch's Letter to the Editor."

15. Culver and Gert, *Philosophy in Medicine: Conceptual and Ethical Issues in Medicine and Psychiatry* (New York: Oxford University Press, 1982), pp. 182-183. Parenthetical remarks added.

16. *Ibid.*, p. 183

17. Marx W. Wartofsky, "Beyond a Whole-Brain Definition of Death: Reconsidering the Metaphysics of Death," in *Death: Beyond Whole-Brain Criteria*, ed. Richard M. Zaner (Dordrecht: Kluwer, 1988), p. 219.

18. President's Commission, p. 11.

19. Rosenberg, *Thinking Clearly About Death.*

20. B. Jennet and F. Plum, "Persistent Vegetative State After Brain Damage," *Lancet*, 1 (1972); David Ingvar *et al.*, "Survival after Severe Cerebral Anoxia with Destruction of the Cerebral Cortex: The Apallic Syndrome," *Annals of the New York Academy of Sciences*, 315 (1978); Ronald Cranford, "The Persistent Vegetative State: The Medical Reality (Getting the Facts Straight)," *Hastings Center Report*, 18 (1988); American Academy of Neurology, "Position Statement of the American Academy of Neurology on Aspects of the Care and Management of the Persistent Vegetative State Patient," *Neurology*, 39 (1989).

Fourteen

DEATH RITUALS IN MALAYSIA: AN EXAMINATION OF THE BELIEFS AND PRACTICES OF CHINESE MALAYSIANS

Anne Eyre

Among the Chinese of the Malaysian Peninsula, a rich cultural heritage has evolved combining Confucianist, Taoist, and Buddhist influences with popular religiosity, superstition, myth, and folklore. Related to this is a series of beliefs and customs associated with preparation for death, disposal of the body, and duty to the ancestors and the spirit world. Ideas about the continuity of life and death (the notion of *samsara*) and the interconnection between the dead and the living re-enforce an emphasis on the proper fulfilment of these ceremonies as necessary both for the successful passage of the soul and for the welfare of the living. Unless regular and appropriate performance of duty to the dead is fulfilled, unpleasant consequences may occur for the living. Thus, merit is accumulated and transferred through pre-mortal and post-mortal customs including arrangements for burial (according to *feng shui*), the performance of elaborate funeral ceremonies, and the burning of "consumer goods" for use by the ancestors in the *yin* world. In the Malaysian context, these customs and beliefs are surviving, adapting to, and accommodating modernistic and secular influences. This is partly because they function to reinforce the heritage and identity of the Chinese in a society of competing ethnic communities.

This chapter focuses on the meaning of death and life for Chinese communities in South East Asia, particularly Chinese Malaysians. Life and death for these people varies vastly from the sort of understanding incorporated in Western secular debates. This is partly because of the traditional religious and cultural context in which death and relationships between persons are set; for example, under the influence of Confucianist ethics, life and death are as much about family and community duties as about individuals. Also, at the popular level, people do not tend to employ academic arguments when it comes to beliefs and rituals associated with life and death; they just do, in the way their ancestors have always done. Consequently, many of our Western philosophical ways of thinking, our questions, and our logic are irrelevant.

T. S. Chee reflects this, describing a similar pattern in Singapore:

> Few Chinese Singaporeans really take a serious intellectual interest in the rituals and rites observed by their community. Almost everything is put under the rubric 'customary.' The practice of rites is dependent on who happens to know something about them and whether their observance complies with 'customary' expectations. There is therefore an overriding indeterminacy.[1]

At the same time, though, I am talking about a part of the world increasingly affected by the sort of modernizing and rationalistic tendencies associated with rapid industrial development, including Western ways of thinking and behavior. One effect of this is that traditional ways of thinking about life and death in South East Asia are themselves evolving and increasingly subject to the same sort of philosophical and ethical lines of questioning seen in the West. Such rationalistic ways of thinking may well in time further modify the beliefs and social customs relating to the dead that I will examine in this chapter.

1. The Chinese in Malaysia

The setting for this chapter is the Chinese communities of West Malaysia (though I will also make references to Singapore). Malaysia has about 14 million inhabitants, of which approximately 40 percent are Chinese. The Chinese started arriving and settling in Malaya as traders from the 1400s but their numbers increased greatly from the 1800s. Indian laborers were also imported by the British, mainly to work on rubber plantations in Malaya. As well as leading to an ethnic and cultural mix which still makes Malaysia a fascinating place to visit today, the pattern of immigration, occupation, and settlement contributed to a society increasingly divided along racial and ethnic lines. As I have argued elsewhere, underlying ethnic conflict has been reinforced by the further demarcation of the races along economic, geographical, political, and religious lines.[2] In this context, the resilience of traditional beliefs and practices among the different ethnic groups is partly explained by its importance in reinforcing communal identity and heritage. We must understand this in order to appreciate the significance of death beliefs and customs as part of wider questions of identity and destiny for the Chinese in Malaysia. Chinese communities are inevitably complex and variable in terms, for example, of regional, dialect, and class distinctions. However, while in this chapter some distinctions, for example between the wealthier and poorer Chinese, are discussed, it tends toward general statements about Chinese traditions. This is not to ignore that within the Chinese community as a whole variation will exist in the extent to which different individuals, families, and communities subscribe to these. Indeed, research such as Chee's (*Religion and Modernisation*) has focussed on the extent to which traditional beliefs and practices are declining over generations and the religious, social consequences of this.

2. Chinese Belief Systems

Before examining death rituals, we must understand the nature of the general religious belief system of the Chinese. Chinese religion is like a jigsaw with many elements drawn from a variety of sources and blended together to make a whole. The three main influences are Confucianism, Taoism, and Buddhism, all of which have blended together as elements in what many scholars refer to as the "Chinese religion."[3] Although aspects of their influence can be identified, it is difficult and, indeed, inappropriate to the popular Chinese mind to try to separate these strands. However, in everyday life, the reverse happens and many regard the three elements as part and parcel of the one religion. "San Chiao Wei Yi" is a popular saying in Hong Kong, meaning "The three religions are one."[4]

> From Buddhism to liberate the soul and become a Buddha; from Taoism to practical meditation as practised by Lao-Tse and eventually the soul will ascend to heaven and become a Buddha; from Confucianism to live virtuously in this world.[5]

Another significant point for understanding Chinese attitudes to life and death is to recognize that Chinese religion is "eminently practical."[6] Beliefs and rituals are "this-worldly." Even beliefs and practices involving the dead are oriented toward success and prosperity of the living. This pragmatic approach is illustrated by the rites of passage that are integrated into the regular celebrations of the wider cycle of life and death in nature.

> Birth, maturation, marriage, old age, and death in the cycle of life are reflected in the planting of spring, growth of summer, harvest of autumn, and old age or rest of winter.[7]

The annual cycle of festivals in the Chinese calendar reflect this cycle of humanity in the cosmos. The festivals relevant here are those commemorating the life and death of ancestors (such as All Souls' Day) as well as those for praying for and appeasing the spirits (such as the Hungry Ghost Festival).

3. Concepts of Life and Death

This cyclical imagery is reflected in the notion of *samsara*—the individual's cycle of birth and death—inherited by Buddhism from its Hindu roots.

> Through reincarnation or rebirth all human beings reap good or evil consequences of their actions. The quality of their deeds of body, their speech, and thought in previous lives determines the circumstances of their rebirth.[8]

"To the Chinese, death is the beginning of another life—the *yin* life."[9] In thinking about death, the Chinese are not thinking so much about finality, as about the continuation of the soul through other stages of life. This idea of the continuity of life and death, and the interconnection between the dead and the living is a central theme of this paper. It reinforces the belief that ceremonies for the deceased have practical implications both for the welfare of the soul as it proceeds along its path and for the living in terms of their consequent fortune and happiness in the present life. The beliefs in ancestor worship and the elaborate courts of hell illustrate this.

4. Ancestor Worship

Ancestor worship is an ancient Chinese custom which has been reinforced by the philosophy and teachings of Confucius (born in 551 BC). His concern was less in religion or questions concerning life and death, and more in the duties of individuals to respect and preserve the institutions of the family and state. A key concept in his writings was "filial piety"—the duty of the individual to attend to the parents. In his *Analects,* he wrote: "When parents are alive, he must serve them according to propriety; and when they die, he must bury them and sacrifice to them according to propriety."[10] It is not a coincidence that Confucius uses exclusive language here; he believed that only males could properly fulfill family duties; hence the practice among generations of Chinese of adopting sons and murdering daughters at birth. This fundamental doctrine of filial piety is reflected in the practice of paying respects to one's ancestors. Every Chinese home and business has altars to gods and ancestors, to whom prayers and offerings are regularly given.

Although Confucius himself was not "religious," ancestor worship (and even the worship of Confucius himself) became a dominant cult among the Chinese and continues throughout the Diaspora. One sinologist, J. Legge, makes a significant point about the meaning of sacrifices to the ancestral spirits. Although referring to imperial state ceremonies as they developed soon after Confucius's time, his point is appropriate today for understanding the meaning and significance of contemporary family ancestor rituals. He says:

> These offerings are oblations, and not sacrifices in our common acceptance of that term. There is not, and never was, any idea of propitiation or expiation in them. They are the tributes of duty and gratitude, accompanied

> with petitions and thanksgivings. They do not express a sense of guilt, but a feeling of dependence.[11]

Mixed in here also are popular beliefs about the presence of the ancestor's spirit/soul which, having left the body at death, possesses the power to incur either good or evil influence over the community. The donation of prayers and offerings are therefore much more than acts of remembrance; they are also aimed at appeasing the souls, inducing them to enter the spirit tablets, and ensuring blessings.

Ancestor worship reflects the Confucian emphasis on duty as a vital element associated with praying to the dead. A second element has also developed within popular Chinese culture based on animist, Buddhist, and Taoist origins. A whole set of mythologies exists associated with gods, spirits, and the heavenly realms around which further death beliefs and rituals have evolved.

5. Heaven and Hell

From popular Mahayana Buddhism comes the idea of a series of realms of existence or worlds, of which the human world is only one. Also existing are the subhuman worlds of ghosts and demons and the heavenly realms—mythically depicted in terms of gardens and palatial beauty as higher places of peace and radiance.

While similarities exist with Judeo-Christian themes, the use of terminology such as "heaven" and "hell" should not be confused with the idea of an eternity, a once and for all passage from which the soul does not move on or return. In keeping with the concept of reincarnation, it would for Buddhists appear to be unreasonable for a person to be condemned to eternal hell on account of their human weakness without being given the chance to redeem themselves. Hell for the Chinese, therefore, is only a temporary punishment, a way of making amends for past deeds as part of the process of preparing for the next incarnation.

A significant concept here for understanding this mobility through the afterlife is the notion of merit. Merit can be thought of as a kind of "credit-debit" account of life. At the point of death, individuals face the mirror of retribution. Here the merits and demerits of their life are weighed against each other and their destiny is determined.

The belief is that those destined to pass through hell can work themselves upwards and outwards by making use of merit accrued either previously or passed on by those still in the human domain. This is the idea of transferring merit which is achieved by doing good and wishing the merit on. An example of a good deed is passing on alms to holy men who will pass on the merit to the departed. Other "meritorious deeds" include community works, like building schools and temples and proper treatment of the ancestors. This leads one writer to say that "there are no locks on the gates of hell. Hell is a temporary place and there is no reason for those beings to suffer there forever."[12]

A way to ease the path through hell is to pass on other worldly currency (hell money) for use on the other side—a means of bribing the guards of the courts of hell according to some legends. This is burned either at the grave side or in temple furnaces provided for the purpose.

Elaborate ideas about the nature of hells have been developed through ancient Chinese myths and stories. They focus on the passage of the soul through the valley of death and the "other-world." One belief is that the prayers carried out by the priest and family during the first seven weeks after death help to influence Yama, the ruler of the courts of justice in the *yin* world to be lenient with the departed soul. This helps to explain why death rituals are long and elaborate.

Evelyn Lip gives an account of the mythology associated with the Ten Courts of Hell.[13] She describes how, having been put in front of the Mirror of Retribution and shown the form of impending reincarnation, the individual proceeds through the other nine courts of justice, each one meting out punishments for types of misdeed, including bribery, tax evasion, cruelty, and drug trafficking.

Details about the number and nature of the differing hells vary according to different sources. Perhaps it is not a coincidence that in Singapore, where drug traffickers are hanged and the authorities attempted to extradite Nick Leeson for corruption, designated hells exist for dealing with these sorts of crimes. This contrasts with the description found in the *Dictionary of Asian Philosophies* which notes only eight hells and marked variations in detail. What is significant for the purposes of this chapter is not so much the detail but that a range of beliefs exists about the passage of the soul after death since this not only reflects moral codes existing in Chinese society but also affects the conduct of funeral rituals and longer term post-funerary customs. Many Chinese would undoubtedly be skeptical about or regard as mere fantasy the details described above, yet would not question the duty to fulfil their obligations to the dead based on these beliefs. So, for example, they would probably not question the practice of calling in Buddhist or Taoist priests after a death to offer prayers and burn incense and paper money.

6. Funeral Customs

Other funeral customs illustrate the belief in the continuation of a person's soul. Traditionally when the body is placed in the coffin, a piece of "other-worldly" currency is placed on the mouth and a fan and twig are placed in each hand to chase away evil spirits.[14] The body of the deceased may be brought back to the home and laid in front of the ancestral altar for several days. At some point, belief holds that the ancestral spirit will enter the tablet placed on the family altar

Features of a Taoist funeral contrast sharply to the dark solemnity of a traditional English send-off. N. Ryan describes the colourful symbolism of the priest's journey into the underworld to trick and cajole the demonic politicians of hell into releasing the soul into paradise:

> Chinese funerals are elaborate affairs, noisy and perhaps ostentatious. But they remain an important part of the Chinese cultural life with its whole emphasis on ensuring that everything is done to make pleasant the existence of the soul after it has departed from their body and from this world. There never can be too much done for the deceased and in fact everything is arranged to ensure that the life of the spirit will be happier than it was on earth.[15]

A mourning period follows the death, when relatives may traditionally wear an armband and/or decline from cutting their hair or nails for seven weeks. They may decide not to engage at all in Chinese New Year celebrations, a noticeable form of self-exclusion since this is regarded as the festive highlight of the year.

An interesting question is whether these alternative conceptions of life and personhood make death less morbid and taboo than in the West. In Britain, traditional taboos are starting to be challenged by developments such as pre-paid funeral plans. We could learn much from Chinese pre-mortal traditions since at the age of sixty it has been customary for people to prepare for death by organizing a coffin and obtaining a burial site. Their children may even present them with "*shou yi*," the clothes they will wear when passing away.[16] In the past, wealthier Chinese belonged to "coffin societies" to which they contributed each month as a way of securing a means of burial. Similar associations based on surname or districts existed for ensuring a place of burial. The procurement of grave clothes and a coffin well before death were traditionally considered symbols of longevity and status.

Another tradition was for the sick to move into what were known as "dying houses" instead of to die at home. Several clan associations and mutual benefit societies ran such outfits. The proprietors would function in a similar way to undertakers, providing all the services for the dead, arranging the funeral and obtaining a hearse, priest and even paid mourners should this be necessary.

Evelyn Lip says that some wealthy Chinese, fearful that their children may not perform all the funeral rites correctly, arrange for their funeral ceremony to be performed while they are still alive. This further reinforces the main theme of this chapter, namely, that the rituals surrounding death are as significant for the deceased and their post-funerary needs as for the bereaved. It gives new meaning to the concept of "do-it-yourself" funerals!

7. Disposal of the Body

In terms of disposing of the body, the most common custom has been burial. Geomancers may be consulted to decide the site and even the time for the burial. This is part of the complex Chinese philosophy relating to *feng shui* according to which the forces of the natural and human environment must be carefully balanced in order to detract evil and increase good fortune. *Feng shui* literally means "wind and water"; it developed from the belief in the forces of *yin* and *yang*, positive and negative. When, by drawing on the principles of *feng shui*, a balance between forces is struck, tranquility and harmony is achieved.[17] Good fortune for the living and the dead will follow. The use of geomancy to balance the *yin* and *yang* forces extends beyond the choice of burial ground to cover other aspects of everyday life such as the design and location of buildings, the arrangement of the furniture within homes and businesses.

Yeoh outlines the historical significance of *feng shui* for the Chinese in Singapore.[18] Its importance was not only in determining the most desirable burial place, but also for guaranteeing reciprocal benefits for the living and the dead. While the dead received veneration, attention and offerings; the living could use their ancestors as mediators for worldly prosperity:

> Geomancy was hence a means through which the Chinese could ...capitalise upon and align themselves to the natural environment in order to appropriate its bounty through the rituals of ancestor worship.[19]

Although today the practice of *feng shui* is limited in Singapore by the few cemetery plots that are left, in Malaysia land is more plentiful and geomancers may still be hired to select good burial sites. According to the practice of *feng shui* a fortuitous place to be buried is on the side of a hill so that the ancestors can have a good view and are protected on one side from evil spirits. Lip explains:

> The burial ground must have the profile of the dragon (rolling hills) and the breath of cosmic life. The Chinese believe that the dead should have good air (*sheng qi*) to breathe. A lack of cosmic breath or good air affects the comfort of the dead and, therefore, the luck of the descendants. Land that is flat, waterlogged or not backed by a hill is considered unsuitable.[20]

Yeoh gives a fascinating account of the use of *feng shui* as a strategic discourse during disputes around the control and location of burial grounds in colonial Singapore at the turn of the twentieth century. When colonial administrators attempted to reclaim the hilly and central burial sites for urban development they soon realized that the concept of government control over burial places was both alien and extremely threatening to the Chinese who wanted the freedom to bury according to *feng shui*. Equally baffling for the Western authorities was the relative priority placed on the dead and the living by the Chinese. To the Western mind, the selection of "the highest and most beautiful sites" for the dead while "the living [dwelt] on the adjacent low swampy ground" with associated health risks was regarded as an incomprehensible inversion.[21] What the Westerners failed to understand was that the place of burial—the *yin* dwelling—is significant because of the belief in the link between the welfare of the dead and the fate of the living.

> Unlike in the west where the habitations of the living and those of the dead belonged to different worlds, in the Chinese view, 'the tomb is the *yin* habitation to match the *yang* habitation of the living' within a single system.[22]

As in other societies, the manner of the disposal of the dead reflects and reinforces class distinctions. In the Chinese context, this is reflected in the type of burial ground, the position of the grave and the nature of the memorial. In colonial Singapore were three types of Chinese burial ground, reflecting class and status distinctions. While some wealthy families had their own private grounds, a second type of burial ground existed for those associated by surname or provenance. The poor would be buried in a third class of grounds open to dialect groups and funded by the wealthier Chinese:

> As in life, the dead were also stratified according to a rigid socio- economic hierarchy and burial places not only symbolized but perpetuated social distinctions which death failed to...eradicate. The principles of unity and lines of cleavage which structured Chinese society in the world of the living were hence equally inscribed and reaffirmed in the sacred spaces of the dead.[23]

While burial is the stronger tradition, cremation (of Buddhist origin) also exists, and today many Malaysian Chinese opt for this. Where urns are stored in pagodas (as opposed to at home or in the ancestral halls of Buddhist temples), what is more desirable and consequently more expensive, is for the cremation urn to be placed higher up the pagoda. In one pagoda I visited such distinctions in economic and social status were marked. The higher one climbed the more elaborate were the urns, the greater the space allocated on the shelf and the more extensive the view from the pagoda's open-style windows.

It follows from the idea of mutual dependence between the living and the dead that favorable disposal is not just a matter of social pride:

> If dead ancestors live in poor conditions, in dampness or badly ventilated areas without *qi* or cosmic breath, the living will also suffer from bad

> fortune or ill health. Therefore it is the duty of the children to attend to the graves of their ancestors, ensuring that the graves are well kept and the spirits comfortable.[24]

Two significant annual festivals in this respect are All Souls' Day and the Hungry Ghost festival.

8. Qing Ming

All Souls' Day, or *Qing Ming* (which means "clean and bright"), is an annual festival which expresses the continuing importance of the Confucian ethic of filial piety. Families visit the graves of their relatives, clean the site, maintain the headstone and offer prayers of gratitude, devotion and remembrance. After tending the grave the family may consume the food offered there.

Popular belief in the presence of the ancestors' spirits means that prayers may also be offered asking for favors or blessings. A common trend is to burn worldly goods for the next life either at the cemetery or in the temple. Tan Teik Beng describes this practice, pointing out at the same time that the practice is not strictly Buddhist:

> Even among those who call themselves Buddhist there still lingers in their minds the possibility that some kind of 'material' heaven exists somewhere in the universe to which their departed ones have been transported at death. Hence, quantities of paper money and other paper objects such as houses, servants, garments, suitcases, motor-cars and even TV sets are transmuted by fire into their spiritual counterparts in the belief that these objects will be enjoyed by the departed ones in the other world.[25]

Beng and Sri Dhammananda stress the futility of these rituals and other emotional displays. All Souls' Day is not meant to be regarded as a sad event in the sense that participants are not mourning an eternal loss. Behavior such as crying is regarded as less appropriate than the sense of satisfaction and peace of mind associated with fulfilling one's duty.

> According to Buddhism, the greatest gift one can give to one's ancestors is to perform meritorious deeds such as giving alms to holy people and printing religious books, and transferring the merits so acquired. Weeping, feeling sorry, lamenting and bewailing at the death of the loved ones are of no benefit to the dead as well as to the living. On the other hand, transferring of merits in this manner not only benefit(s) the departed ones, but those who perform it also receive the fruits of their deed.[26]

Such charitable deeds also function to benefit the community in general and reinforce the status of the holy men as mediators of merit. Thus the interests of those writing on behalf of the Buddhist Missionary Society, such as Beng and Sri Dhammananda, are best served in stressing this tradition.

9. Hungry Ghost Festival

The Hungry Ghost Festival has both Buddhist and Taoist origins. It rests on the superstition that during the seventh month the souls of the dead are released from hell on vacation and wander the earth intermingling with the living. Some are sad spirits because families have neglected to honor them; they have an insatiable craving for offerings which will grant them acceptance and peace. Throughout this month, priests and the public burn joss sticks and paper money. They make abundant offerings of food and wine in order to appease these spirits and seek benevolent favors in return. Hungry ghosts may be vengeful (if they died suddenly for example), and the function of prayers and offerings is also to mitigate against their anger and ensure their return to the other-world after the vacation period. Lip describes how in more elaborate ceremonies an effigy of *Yama* may be made and a roasted pig's head may be placed in front of the effigy.[27]

Much superstition exists among the Chinese about wandering spirits. Many will opt not to marry or make unnecessary journeys during this time and accidents or illness may be attributed to the work of ghosts. In Chinese films, stories reflecting such widespread superstitions about the spirit world abound. One, for example, features the incarnation of a ghost in the form of a pretty woman whose disguise deceives innocent young men until a priest is employed to send the spirit back to hell and restore order.

10. Conclusion: The Encounter with Modernity

This chapter has illustrated how Chinese beliefs and practices surrounding mortality reflect cyclical notions of life and death. This provides an alternative perspective to Western philosophical approaches which attempt to demarcate more precise distinctions between life and death.

At the same time, however, the Chinese are facing ethical dilemmas and social questions associated with death and dying that are raised by the impact of modernity. Burial ground in Singapore is fast running out, the proportion of dependent elderly people is growing rapidly, and in the pace of modern life the younger generation is becoming more mobile, secular, and discerning of tradition. In Malaysia—one of the fastest growing economies of the world—will these centuries-old traditions die out in the next millennium?

Sociological evidence regarding religion and postmodernism suggests that this will not necessarily be so. While in the future individuals and communities may well exercise more choice with regard to religious thought and practice, what is unlikely is that they will reject them wholesale. At the same time, and in keeping with historical patterns of adaptation and inculturation, Chinese beliefs, superstitions, and rituals will probably continue to incorporate features of modernity and reflect the needs of contemporary economic life.

For example, at today's funerals and on All Souls' Day, not only might hell money be burned but also cardboard replicas of modern consumer goods such as American Express cards, cheque books, televisions, videos, hair-dryers, mobile phones, cans of beer, cigarettes, and jewelry. All of these will be burned in order to enable the deceased to prosper in a similar manner to that which they have been accustomed in life.

A further reason why Chinese traditions are likely to survive in Malaysia relates to the observations made at the beginning of this chapter. In a society of competing ethnic identities, the history and heritage of the Chinese is being preserved through its death rituals and cycle of festivals. In this way, commemoration and remembrance function for the present and the future as much as for the past.

NOTES

1. T.S. Chee, *Religion and Modernisation: A Study of Changing Rituals Among Singapore's Chinese, Malays, and Indians* (Singapore: Graham Brash, 1985), p. 64.

2. Anne Eyre, "Religion, Politics, and Development in Malaysia," in R.H. Roberts ed., *Religion and the Transformations of Capitalism* (London: Routledge, 1995).

3. Chee, *Religion and Modernisation*, p. 6.

4. Bloomfield Frena, *The Book of Chinese Beliefs* (London: Arrow Books, 1983), p. 39.

5. N. J. Ryan, *The Cultural Heritage of Malaya* (Malaysia: Longman, 1971), p. 97.

6. M. Saso, "Chinese Religions," in J. Hinnells ed., *A Handbook of Living Religions* (Harmondsworth: Penguin Books, 1984), p. 354.

7. *Ibid.*, p. 354.

8. R. Drummond, "The Buddha's Teaching," in *A Lion Handbook: The World's Religions* (Oxford: Lion Publishing, 1988), p. 231.

9. Evelyn Lip, *Chinese Beliefs and Superstitions* (Singapore: Graham Brash, 1985), p. 1.

10. Confucius, *Analects* in D.H. Smith, *Confucius* (St. Albans: Paladin, 1973), p. 73.

11. James Legge, *The Religion of China* (London: Hodder and Stoughton, 1880), p. 53.

12. Ven Dr K Sri Dhammananda, *What Buddhists Believe* (Malaysia: Buddhist Missionary Society, 1987), p. 303.

13. Lip, *Chinese Beliefs*, pp. 11-15.

14. *Ibid.*, p. 22.

15. N. Ryan, *The Cultural Heritage of Malaya*, pp. 123-124.

16. Lip, *Chinese Beliefs*, p. 22.

17. *Ibid.*, p. 79.

18. B. Yeoh, "The Control of 'Sacred' Space: Conflicts over the Chinese Burial Grounds in Colonial Singapore, 1880-1930," *Journal of Southeast Asian Studies*, 22:2 (September 1991), pp. 282-311.

19. *Ibid.*, p. 298.

20. Evelyn Lip, *Chinese Temples and Deities* (Singapore: Times Books International, 1986), p. 44.

21. Yeoh, "The Control of Sacred Space," p. 287.

22. *Ibid.*, p. 310.

23. *Ibid*, pp. 300-301.

24. Lip, *Chinese Beliefs*, p. 32.

25. Tan Teik Beng, *Beliefs and Practices Among Malaysian Chinese Buddhists* Kuala Lumpur: Buddhist Missionary Society, 1988), pp. 52-53.

26. *Ibid.*, p. 52.

27. Lip, *Chinese Beliefs*, p. 74.

Fifteen

BECOMING PERSONAL: A LIBERATIVE THEOLOGICAL PERSPECTIVE

Andrew Dawson

The following chapter explores the concept of person as it is held by thinkers within the school of Latin-American liberation theology. As the liberationist understanding of what it means to be a person is developed, themes and preoccupations articulated by European personalist thinkers will constantly come to the fore.[1] This should be no surprise as the indebtedness of Latin-American liberation theology to the European personalist tradition is readily acknowledged by key liberation theologians.[2] The structures of Catholic Action, research movements headed by people such as Louis Lebret and François Houtart, the influence of the New Theology, and seminary education in Europe, each gave impetus to the Latin-American reception of the emerging themes and chief preoccupations of the personalist movement.[3]

Furthermore, the favorable reception of personalist concerns in Latin America should be no surprise, given the common intellectual framework of the Roman Catholic social teaching. Initiated in the modern era by the papal encyclicals *Rerum Novarum* (1891) and *Quadragesimo Anno* (1931), the Roman Catholic tradition of social commentary carefully charted a middle way between the two prevailing extremes of capitalist liberal individualism and state-communist collectivism.[4] The later encyclicals of *Mater et magistra* (1961) and *Pacem in terris* (1963) did much to facilitate the transmission of a personalist agenda to Latin America. We may claim for the personalist and liberationist traditions a significant role in the development of Roman Catholic social concerns for political and socio-economic rights.

As many nuances and differences exist in emphasis among Latin-American liberation theologians, this chapter represents no more than a series of broad brush strokes upon an extensive canvas. Nevertheless, a sufficient degree of common ground exists within the liberationist school so as to allow a representative picture to be drawn of its concept of the person. This common ground upon which all liberation theologians stand is constituted by what they regard as an "integral," we might say "holistic," concept of the person. Two points by way of clarification.

1. The Integral Person

First, in theological terms, liberation theology fundamentally rejects the traditional distinction between the orders of Creation and Redemption; that is, the belief that God affects the salvation of humankind by means which are other than historically realizable and practicably concrete. The realms of the supernatural and the natural are thereby conjoined by liberation theology, elided within one and the same historical process. For liberation theology, then, no such thing as a "pure nature" exists which has not already been touched by divine grace. God is intrinsically immersed in the warp and woof of everyday existence. No historical reality exists which does not, in some way, bear the marks of its divine origins.

In tandem with its historical unification of the realms of the supernatural and the natural, liberation theology likewise articulates a unified, psycho-physical concept of the person. Exemplified by the paradigm of the Incarnation, the ongoing historical process of divine immersion finds its consummate unification in the holistic, integral concept of the person. As no historical reality exists which is not touched by the machinations of divine grace, no talk of God working upon a spiritual soul in isolation from the physical body can occur.[5] Consequently, any theological description of the person which articulates a concept of the soul as recognizably discontinuous with the body is rejected as an arcane form of dualism.[6] For liberation theologians, the person does not have a soul, the person is embodied soul; that is, a living, psycho-physical unity which bears testimony to the saving activity of God in history.

Second, in anthropological terms, liberation theology works with a decentred concept of the person. Although the term "decentred" is more readily employed by post-modern social theorists (for example, Foucault, Ricoeur) than by liberation theologians, it serves well to emphasize the liberationist concern to de-individualize all talk of personal existence. Liberation theology rejects traditional theological (for example, Boethius, Anselm) and modern liberal (Rousseau, early Sartre, Novak) conceptualizations of the subject as social isolate whose personhood is a pre-constituted fact. Whether in traditional or modern guise, personal atomism runs counter to the liberationist view that we are never discrete individuals whose personhood is attained in isolation from other factors. To exist is to be located, and to be located is to be situated amidst a plethora of interpenetrative determinisms. In becoming personal, the human subject engages with a plurality of bodily, historical and social phenomena. Each of these phenomena, in a wide variety of ways, constitutes the environment within which the individual attains personhood in relation to others.[7] Within liberation theology, the person is always person-as-related-to-another.

The intersection of the theological and anthropological axes of liberation theology's integral understanding of person-as-related-to-another is seen nowhere more clearly than in its concept of "salvation as liberation." Given the unification of history and the decentred concept of personal existence, salvation ceases to be articulated in terms of a private and internalized elevation of the soul from a natural to a supernatural plane. Instead, an integral concept of the person demands an integral concept of salvation. The concept of salvation is thereby historicized and decentred by liberation theologians:

> Salvation does not take shape, therefore, as a reality beyond the world, to be reached only *post*-history, in the life of the hereafter. Instead, it begins to be realized here. Though still not fully consummated, eternal life is already given to us by the Son of God in the here and now of human life...irrupting within the fabric of human history, being revealed in the long and complex process of human liberation.[8]

Although careful not to undermine the transcendent dimension and post-historical fulfillment of God's saving activity, it is to underline the historical and decentred nature of salvation that the term "liberation" is utilized. Talk of salvation as liberation, then, means that in being saved, humanity is not saved from history, but saved within and for the sake of history. As Hugo Assmann puts it, the history of salvation is "the salvation of history."[9]

2. Becoming Personal

The use of the term "liberation" as shorthand for an historicized and decentred conception of salvation is founded upon an understanding of people as those who exist at all times in relation to someone or something other than themselves. Consequently, the word "person" stands always as a shorthand rendering of person-as-related-to-another. At the same time, we must not lose sight that all relations with the other (whomever or whatever it might be) occur within a particular psycho-physical, historical, and social setting. Personal existence is situated existence. So, in addition to the above rejection of an individualized conceptualization of the person, liberation theology likewise refuses to countenance an overly abstruse and ahistorical account of human subjectivity (for example, Kant). Holding these thoughts in view, the following pages elucidate a liberationist perspective upon what it means to become personal. In short, I seek to make the claim that we are liberated only to the extent that we become persons; yet we become persons only to the extent that we participate in relations with others in a truly liberative (that is historicized and decentred) manner.

To facilitate a liberative understanding of what it means to become personal, the concept of person-as-related-to-another will be examined by way of a tripartite analytical framework comprising the intrapersonal, the interpersonal and the transpersonal dimensions of human existence. Each of these three dimensions represents a nuanced way of conceptualizing the person-as-related-to-another. As such, the intrapersonal (microscopic) dimension concerns itself with a theological articulation of person-constituting relations at a non-public level; the interpersonal (mesoscopic) dimension focuses upon the communal level of person-to-person relations; while the transpersonal (macroscopic) dimension comprises an examination of person-forming relations as they are mediated through historical and societal structures. I will note from the outset, however, that each of these dimensions is separated from the other two solely by means of reflective abstraction for the purposes of analytical clarity. In actuality, each of these dimensions of personal existence is penetrated by and dependent upon the others for its fullest expression. As all three dimensions are mutually constituted and reciprocally constituting in their relations, no representative picture of personal becoming can be drawn which does not include reference to each one.

A. Intrapersonal Dimension

Within the intrapersonal dimension of personal becoming, the formal object of the self is the "Absolute Other" whom the Christian religion has come to know as God. Although no consensus exists in liberation theology as to the extent and manner of humankind's natural orientation toward the Absolute Other, widespread agreement exists that the presence and activity of God serves as the ultimate foundation of all human experience.[10] God's involvement as the primordial and constitutive (that is ontological) base of all subsequent personal becoming is recognized at a conscious (that is existential) level by way of faith. Comprising the acknowledgement of our absolute dependence as persons upon a personal God, faith both informs our reading of the world around us and impels us to personalize this world by way of practical engagement with it.[11]

The Absolute Other, however, is not only the foundation of all human experience. As the person in all of his historical concreteness "is destined to communion with God," God is present to us also as the Transcendent Other; that is, the goal, the end of all human striving.[12] Utilizing the classical definition of the Trinity as a "community of persons," liberation theologians regard humankind as being called to "participate" within the Divine "society."[13] The perichoretic harmony of the Trinity constitutes a community of divine persons which is at all times open to the participation of each human person. Although of a primarily private nature, the intrapersonal dimension of human existence is nevertheless a social affair; a social affair in which the Transcendent Other is encountered as a community of persons, and human personhood enhanced by means of inclusion within the Divine life. The more we respond to God's call to become the other (that is, better) person that God would have us be, the more we are included within the personalizing dynamic of the divine life. Initiated by the prevenient activity of God as the absolute foundation of all personal existence, personhood is nevertheless enhanced by the assumption of individual responsibility for who we are and what we might become.

Although never shying away from exploring the intrapersonal dimension of human existence as a relationship with the Transcendent Other, liberation theology is at constant pains to avoid an uncritical privatization of human religiosity. In developing a "spirituality of liberation," Latin-American theologians have highlighted the wholesale "interiorization" to which our personal relations with God have been subjected within the Christian tradition.[14] Liberation theology maintains that tradition's concern with the private, "vertical" dimension of God–human relations have resulted in the subjugation of the public, "horizontal" dimension of the Christian faith.[15] For this reason, whenever liberation theology describes salvation as "the communion of human beings with God", it does so by adding "and among themselves."[16] For liberation theology, God is encountered not only as the ground and end of my being, but also in the concrete, visible face of my neighbor. Within the internally oriented dynamic by which God is experienced as foundation and goal of personal existence, a complementary centrifugal dynamic is contained through which the personal subject is impelled to seek communion with other persons. This affirmation leads us to consider the second (mesoscopic) dimension of human existence, the interpersonal.

B. Interpersonal Dimension

The interpersonal dimension of human existence is constituted by the tangible presence of a visible other who is my neighbor. Upon being confronted with the limitless possibilities of direct, face-to-face relations with another human being, the person encounters a public domain which demands either affirmation or rejection. Any neutral, third way of indifference (*apatheia*) to the visible other who is my neighbor can never exist. Christian love (*agape*), is translated as "solidarity" by theologians of liberation, and solidarity requires both a recognition of the other as independent of myself and an acceptance of the obligations which the freedom and equality of the other impose upon me as their neighbor.[17]

The cause of solidarity is never allowed by liberation theology to spill over into an uncritical homogenization in which individuality and difference are subsumed within a superficial sameness. The theistic metaphysics and universalist anthropology of liberation theology make for an easy affirmation of our "common humanity."[18] At the same time, however, it is strongly affirmed that true personhood is realized by "the one who achieves a balance between autonomy and communion, solitude and fusion."[19] Within the interpersonal dimension of human existence, personhood flourishes at that mid-point which stands between the two poles of individualism and massification. The extreme of individualism is countered by the constant struggle for solidarity, while the excesses of collectivism are neutralized by the ongoing affirmation of difference.[20]

Solidarity with and difference from the visible other are best guarded from the excesses of atomism and homogeneity by the formation of community. For liberation theology, no meaningful talk of personal existence exists which does not make explicit reference to the impact which community has upon any particular individual. As Comblin maintains, "there is no such thing as a person apart from community."[21] To be personal is to be in community; to be a person, is to be related-to-another. Whether in the primary community of kinship structures or in the secondary community of the work-place, for example, it is in the face-to-face encounter with other human beings that personhood is most facilitated and enriched. "The essence of the Christian life," "Christianity's contribution" to the liberation of the world, and humanity's "response to God's call" all lie in the formation of community as the arena for personal becoming.[22]

Within the face-to-face encounter of community, others are experienced for what and who they are. The tangible presence of the visible other before me inhibits any false projection on my part in which the other is constructed out of the matrix of my wishes, preoccupations, and personal prejudices. In standing before me in the act of community, the visible other challenges the stereotypes by which I seek to define and thereby delimit his personhood. Authentic community both transcends simplistic appeals to sameness which subvert the challenge of my neighbor's difference from me and demands that this difference not be allowed to obscure an appreciation of those things we hold in common. No mere coincidence exists that liberation theology has found such a rich source of stimulating material in the concrete experience of the base ecclesial movement in Latin America, a movement which is predicated upon the fructification of personhood within a context of Christian solidarity with the visible other. The base ecclesial community constitutes a fertile womb within which the daily lessons of interpersonal encounter furnish liberation theologians with a lived experience which daily attests to the importance of "intimate participation... direct relationships...reciprocity...mutual assistance...[and] communality."[23] Intimacy, reciprocity and mutuality, such are the mediations by which face-to-face relations are constituted as a sphere of person making.

A further contribution of the base ecclesial community to the maturation of liberation theology has been the manner in which it has grounded theological reflection in the concrete experience of the day-to-day struggles of the masses.[24] A constant refrain of liberation theologians reminds the theological community in the North of the difference between their respective theoretical problematics. The northern community is believed to have a predilection for asking how it might speak of God in an age of unbelief. For liberation theology, however, the issue is not one of secularization, but that of reflecting upon the personalizing affirmations of the faith in a society which is thoroughly dehumanizing.[25] Rooted in the daily experiences of the impoverished majority, liberation theology is never allowed to reflect upon the person as some abstract phenomenon divorced from the concrete realities of existence. Human existence is always situated existence; the visible other is always encountered as one who is embedded within a given historical, social, economic, political, and cultural milieu.[26]

As personal existence is situated existence, Christian love—solidarity with the other—can never be blind, it is instead "love for the other in view of that other's own reality."[27] The visible other is met as one who is poor, one who is black, one who is female, one who is a Serb, Croat, or Muslim. Consequently, true love for the other comprises both the affirmation of solidarity, in that infinite value transcends all plurality, and the acknowledgement of difference, in that we are each encountered as male or female, black or white, rich or poor, Protestant or Catholic. Authentic community among persons, *koinonia*, is "communion with diversity."[28]

These reflections upon the person as one who is embedded within a given historical and societal matrix bring us to the third dimension of human existence, that of the transpersonal.

C. Transpersonal Dimension

In reflections upon the transpersonal (macroscopic) nature of human existence liberation theology makes perhaps its greatest contribution to the personalist tradition. Within the transpersonal dimension of human existence, the formal object of the self is what can be termed the invisible other, the one who is "distant from me."[29] The term "invisible other" is used to underline the indirect, oblique nature of person-to-person relations within the transpersonal dimension of human existence. Here, the face of the other is not directly before me. Who and what the other is for me is not communicated by the tangible presence of the visible other whose personhood is experienced in the immediacy of interpersonal encounter. Instead, the effect of my actions upon the other, and the other's actions upon me, are mediated by any number of historical, economic, political, social, and cultural matrices.

Within the transpersonal dimension of human existence, societal relations are channeled by objective structures, instead of taking place at the level of subjective, intentionally directed encounters. The indirect and structurally mediated nature of these relations facilitate the fabrication and proliferation of stereotypes and representations which ultimately obscure and pervert the true identity of the other. In obfuscating the reality of who the invisible other is for me, these stereotypes and representations leave the invisible other open to an unfounded rejection and subsequently serve as the justification for her exploitation. An example commonly cited by theologians of liberation is that of the post-discovery depersonalization of the indigenous peoples of South America which made way for their subsequent repression at the hands of newly arrived Europeans.[30] Contemporary instances can be drawn from the use of sexual, racial, and ethnic stereotypes as a means to defining and ultimately channeling the life chances of those categorized under one heading or another.[31]

The objective structures and mechanisms through which the invisible other is represented to me are never the result of conscious or intended activity. From the shop I buy my clothing to the supermarket from which I purchase my groceries, the jokes I tell or laugh at in the street to the magazines and newspapers I read, from the bank which manages my account to the political party I vote for, each of these avenues of daily living mediates and transposes into the prevailing life-world the practical options I make. Generated initially by human activity, these structures and world views nevertheless assume over time an objective (and often unintended) existence, subsequently enduring with an autonomy of their own.

The transpersonal dimension of human existence unfolds within a societal arena constituted by a plurality of conflicting world-views and competing structural processes. Mediated by way of, for example, class relations, inter-racial tension, sexual discrimination, and internecine ethnic strife, such transpersonal processes serve to pit person against person on the grounds of difference and otherness. Thus, while many individuals go through life not counting themselves as racist, sexist, or ethnically prejudiced, for example, the transpersonal *ethos* or structural processes within which they exist may well induce them to act in ways which, intentioned or not, ultimately result in consequences injurious to the personal becoming of others. In effect, the transpersonal dimension of human existence comprises structures and processes which, directly or tangentially, generate requirements and facilitate actions through which the infinite value of the other is either obscured or perverted. In both cases the moral demands of personhood are lost, and the other, by way of spatial or epistemic distance, is rendered practically invisible. Hence, the invisible other obtains.

Those structures and processes which encourage or facilitate the obfuscation of personhood at a transpersonal dimension, liberation theology regards as sinful. For example, if sin is manifest at the intrapersonal level as an ignoring of the call of God, and at the interpersonal level as the breakdown of face-to-face relations, sin is manifest at the transpersonal level by means of unjust structures. Social or structural sin has for decades been a key component of the liberationist articulation of the transpersonal dimension of human existence.[32] I do not mean to suggest that the unjust structures themselves do the sinning. Instead, unjust structural conditions such as poverty, hunger, exploitation, oppression, racism, sexism, and all forms of bigotry and inequality generate a social context in which sin is objectified and the person placed in an environment which facilitates and propagates selfishness, prejudice, ignorance, ambivalence, and other forms of injurious dispositions and actions. As Comblin maintains:

> Personal sins do not occur in isolation. They do not proceed merely from individual wills. Quite the contrary, personal sins also proceed from social and cultural contexts. No one is forced to sin; but cultural and social conditions are such that sin becomes, as it were, normal and easy. While someone is personally responsible for individual sins, these sins are also bound up with situations of sin—tied to social, structural sin.[33]

Individual responsibility is not ignored; it is, however, mitigated with reference to the situated nature of personal becoming. The relationship between individual and structural sin is dialectical in nature; "they mutually strengthen and feed off each other."[34]

In explicating the transpersonal dimension of human existence, liberation theology has decentred sin and thereby posited salvation—as the overcoming of sin—not only as an intrapersonal phenomenon, but also as a "social and historical reality."[35] As "there is no such thing as a religious sin that is not a political and economic sin—and vice versa," no remedy for sin can exist which is not also transpersonal in nature.[36]

Structural sin finds its nemesis in "structural grace."[37] Structural grace is a term used by liberation theologians to designate God's love for the world as it is mediated through historical structures which strive to combat the realities of social sin. For liberation theology, such structures of grace find their ultimate expression in a preferential option for the poor. Sacramental participation is a structure of grace, as are the base ecclesial communities or any other form of socially organized activity which enhances personal becoming in all of its dimensions. However, while serving as a structure of grace, such structures never cease to be historical mediations and so remain at all times "imperfect," "ambivalent," "partial," "ambiguous," and "relative" (that is, open to the effects of sin).[38]

Emerging from the above recognition, liberation theologians refuse to reify any one political party, economic system, or mode of activism over and against others. The primary issue is not which political party must be followed or which economic system adopted. Instead, the principal preoccupation of liberation theology concerns which practical means will best effect the desired end of a social structure in which sin and its effects can be fought. Those options which are chosen or recommended are done so solely on the basis that these means represent the most effective available route, given the historical and social circumstances, to the desired end of a person-making society. No economic, political, or ideological system stands as an end in itself. Instead, such structures are valued only to the extent that they mediate grace in the battle against all depersonalizing historical and social phenomena. The measure against which liberation theology evaluates every potential medium of divine grace is the theological concept of the "reign of God". It is with brief reference to the reign of God that this chapter concludes.

3. Conclusion

Given the unification of history and the de-centering of the concepts of sin, grace, and salvation, the eschatological motif of the reign of God is brought to bear as a tangible, historical reality by which every liberative practice is to be measured.[39] Although the reign of God stands as a tangible, historical phenomenon, it is a reality that will not be fully consummated until the *dénouement* of the created order itself.[40] Dependent for its gradual, yet always partial, realization in history upon the efforts of humankind to construct a more personalizing world, the reign of God comprises the complete affirmation of the person in every dimension of human existence. As the herald of the reign of God, Jesus's life, death, and resurrection constitute a paradigm in which those struggling for the cause of personal becoming might find encouragement and strength.[41]

Whether at an intrapersonal, interpersonal, or transpersonal level, any disposition or action which enhances the capability for personhood is a partial contribution toward the unfolding of the reign of God in history. Initiated by humankind's co-operation with the underlying presence of God, activities as diverse as private contemplation, communal prayer, individual stands for justice, collective action for peace, and every kind of corporate struggle for a better world serve to liberate humanity in every dimension from the depersonalizing effects of sin. To be saved is to be liberated, to be liberated is to become personal, to become personal is to participate fully in the historical growth of the reign of God.

NOTES

1. *E.g.*, Jacques Maritain, *Scholasticism and Politics*, 2nd edition (London: Centenary Press, 1945), pp. 45-70. Emmanuel Mounier, *Personalism* (London: University of Notre Dame Press, 1952), pp. 3-16.

2. *E.g.*, Jose Comblin, *Being Human: A Christian Anthropology* (Kent: Burns & Oates, 1990), p. 51. Enrique Dussel, *Ethics and Community* (Kent: Burns & Oates, 1988), p. 238.

3. Lima A. G. de Souza, *A JUC: Os Estudantes Católicos e a Política* (Petrópolis: Editora Vozes, 1984), p. 175. Eduardo Hoornaert, "Os Três fatores da Nova Hegemonia Dentro da Igreja Católica no Brasil: Fatos e Perspectivas," *Revista Ecclesiástica Brasileira* (1986), pp. 373-374.

4. John A. Coleman., "Neither Liberal nor Socialist: The Originality of Catholic Social Teaching," in John A. Coleman, *One Hundred Years of Catholic Social Thought: Celebration and Challenge* (New York: Orbis, 1991), pp. 25-42.

5. Jose Comblin, "Grace," in Jon Sobrino and Ignacio Ellacuría, *Mysterium Liberationis: Fundamental Concepts of Liberation Theology* (New York, Orbis, 1993) p. 522.

6. Ignacio Ellacuría, "The Historicity of Christian Salvation," in Sobrino and Ellacuría, *Mysterium Liberationis*, p. 522.

7. Leonardo Boff, *Teologia do Cativeiro a da Libertaçã* (Lisbon: Multinova, 1975), pp. 20-23.

8. Lima A. G. de Souza, *Evolução Política dos Católicos e da Igreja no Brasil: Hipóteses para uma Interpretação* (Petropolis: Editora Vozes, 1979), pp. 194-195.

9. Hugo Assman, *Teología desde de la Praxis de la Liberación: Ensayo Telógico desde la América Dependiente*, 2nd edition (Salamanca: Ediciones Sígueme, 1976), p. 25.

10. *E.g.*, Jose Comblin, "Grace," p. 530 and Ignatio Ellacuría, "The Historicity of Christian Salvation," in Sobrino and Ellacuría, *Mysterium Liberationis*, p. 277. Antonio Moser and Bernardino Leers, *Moral Theology: Dead Ends and Ways Forward* (Kent: Burns & Oates, 1990), p. 135. Jon Sobrino, "Spirituality and the Following of Jesus," in Sobrino Ellacuría, *Mysterium Liberationis*, p. 685.

11. Leonardo Boff, "Epistemology and Method of the Theology of Liberation," in Sobrino and Ellacuría, *Mysterium Liberationis*, p. 59. Boff, *Teologia* pp. 30-33.

12. Gustavo Gutiérrez, *A Theology of Liberation: History, Politics, and Salvation*, 2nd edition (London: SCM, 1988), p. 113. Cf. Augustine, *Confessions*, I,i. Aquinas, *Summa Theologiae*, Ia, 8, 3

13. Leonardo Boff, *The Trinity and Society* (Kent: Burns & Oates, 1988).

14. Pedro Casaldáliga and Jose Maria Vigil, *The Spirituality of Liberation* (Kent: Burns & Oates, 1994), pp. 103-110.

15. Juan Luis Segundo, *Evolution & Guilt* (Dublin: Gill & Macmillan, 1980), p. 63.

16. Gutiérrez, *A Theology of Liberation*, p. 113.

17. Casaldáliga and Vigil, *The Spirituality of Liberation*, pp. 103-110. Comblin, *Being Human* p. 12.

18. Moser, and Leers, *Moral Theology*, p. 147.

19. Comblin, *Being Human*, p. 95.

20. *Ibid.*, pp. 10-14.

21. *Ibid.*, p. 95.

22. Dussel, *Ethics and Community*, p. 7. Comblin, *Being Human*, p. 3. Moser and Leers, *Moral Theology*, p. 132.

23. Leonardo Boff, *Ecclesiogenesis: The Base Communities Reinvent the Church* (London: Collins, 1986), p. 4.

24. A. Alonso, *Communidades Eclesiales de Base: Teologí-Sociología-Pastoral* (Salamanca: Ediciones Sigueme, 1970), pp. 239-260. Carlos Mesters, *Defence!ess Flower: A New Reading of the Bible* (New York: Orbis, 1989), pp. 55-155.

25. Gustavo Guitérrez, *The Power of the Poor in History* (New York: Orbis, 1983), p. 92.

26. Gutiérrez, *A Theology of Liberation*, p. 113.

27. Dussel, *Ethics and Community*, p. 10.

28. Jose Ignacio Gonzalez Faus,"Anthropology: The Person and the Community," in Sobrino and Ellacuría, *Mysterium Liberationis*, p. 504.

29. Gustavo Gutiérrez, "Introduction: Liberation, Theology and Proclamation," in Hugo Assmann, *Practical Theology of Liberation* (London: Search Press, 1975), p. 7.

30. Eduardo Hoornaert, "Primeiro Período: A Evangelização do Brasil Durante a Primeira Época Colonial," in J. H. Rodrigues *História da Igreja no Brasil: Ensaio de Interpretação a Partir do Povo* (São Paulo: Edições Paulinas), pp. 142-152.

31. Branadão and Tepedino, "Women and the Theology of Liberation," in Sobrino and Ellacuría, *Mysterium Liberationis*, pp. 223-226. P. Richard, *et al.*, "Challenges to Liberation Theology in the Decade of the Nineties," in Guillermo Cook, *New Face of the Church in Latin America* (New York: Orbis, 1994), pp. 249-250.

32. Casaldáliga and Vigil, *The Spirituality of Liberation*, pp. 156-157. Dussel, *Ethics and Community*, pp. 20-26. Ellacuría, "The Historicity of Christian Salvation," in Sobrino and Ellacuría, *Mysterium Liberationis*, pp. 263, 275. Gutiérrez, *A Theology of Liberation*, p. 103.

33. Comblin, *Being Human*, p. 219. See also Sobrino, "Central Position," p. 355.

34. Casaldáliga, Vigil, *The Spirituality of Liberation*, p. 157.

35. Gutiérrez, *A Theology of Liberation*, pp. 100-101.

36. Dussel, *Ethics and Community*, p. 26.

37. Ellacuría, "The Historicity of Christian Salvation," in Sobrino and Ellacuría, *Mysterium Liberationis*, pp. 263, 276. Segundo Galilea, *The Way of Living Faith: A Spirituality of Liberation* (London: Harper & Row, 1988), pp. 67-71.

38. Comblin, *Being Human* pp. 34-35. Casaldáliga and Vigil, *The Spirituality of Liberation*, p. 177.

39. Sobrino, "Central Position of the Reign of God in Liberation Theology," in Sobrino and Ellacuría, *Mysterium Liberationis*, p. 352.

40. Comblin, *Being Human*, p. 220. Dussel, *Ethics and Community*, p. 15. Sobrino,"Central Position" pp. 360, 372, 382.

41. Sobrino, "Central Position," p. 352. Leonardo Boff, *Jesus Christ Liberator: A Critical Christology of Our Time* (London: SPCK, 1980), pp. 69-75.

ABOUT THE EDITORS AND CONTRIBUTORS

H. Mike Awalt, Belmont University, USA. Awalt has been Professor of Philosophy at Belmont University since 1970. He did his undergraduate work at Baylor University, earned a M.Div. from Southwestern Baptist Theological Seminary, and received his Ph.D. from Baylor University. His specializations include: Existentialism and Phenomenology, Postmodernism, Kierkegaard, Nietzsche, and Philosophy of Film. He received the Award for Innovative Excellence in Teaching, Learning, and Technology from the National Conference on College Teaching and Learning, won the Ernest L. Boyer International Award for Excellence in Teaching, Learning and Technology, and received the Chaney Distinguished Professor Award at Belmont University.

Chris Belshaw, The Open University, Manchester, UK. Belshaw studied philosophy at the University of York, and later at the University of California, Santa Barbara. He has taught at both institutions, as well as at St. Martin's College (Lancaster) and Lancaster University, joining the Open University as Arts Staff Tutor in 1994. His current concerns are with the theoretical side of applied ethics: questions of the value of death, the nature of a person, and related questions in aesthetics and metaphysics.

Matthew Bonzo, Cornerstone University, USA. Bonzo has been an Assistant Professor of Philosophy and Religion at Cornerstone University since 1998. He received a B.S. from Liberty University in 1986, and an M.A. from Trinity Evangelical Divinity School in 1991. He received his Ph.D. from Vrije Universiteit, Amsterdam

Charles C. Conti, University of Sussex, UK. Conti is a Lecturer in Philosophy at the School of English & American Studies at the University of Sussex. His areas of interest include the interdisciplinary links between literature, philosophy, and theology. He started two international philosophical organizations: The Society for the Study of the Philosophical Theology of Austin Farrer and The Personalist Forum. He is the author of *Metaphysical Personalism* (1995). His articles have appeared in journals such as *The Personalist Forum* and *Modern Theology.*

Tony Dancer, Queen's College, Oxford, UK. Dancer lives and works in Oxford, where he has studied theology for a number of years. He is committed to teaching and developing theological education and ministry that is concerned with the ongoing formation of ethical, moral, and personal identity. He is currently completing a doctorate examining the life and work of William Stringfellow. He recently organized the highly successful international conference on Stringfellow; the book that arose from that conference is forthcoming.

Andrew Dawson, University College, Chester, UK. Dawson received a BA with Honors from Manchester University, England, in Theology. He was a World Council of Churches Scholar at the Chicago Theological Seminary. And he received his D.Phil. from the University of Oxford as a British Academy Scholar. He is currently the Senior Lecturer in Contemporary Theologies at Chester College. His areas of research include Contemporary Social and Political Theologies, Christian Social Ethics, and Latin American Studies. He is the author of *The Emergence and Impact of the Base Ecclesial Community and Liberative Theological Discourse in Brazil* (1999).

Peter A. Day, Chipping Norton, UK. Day's main area of interest is early church and Patristic theology, with an emphasis on the work of Origen of Alexandria. His recent focus has been on concepts of universal salvations within Christianity and their influence on Theodicy. Day is currently completing a doctoral thesis on Origen and universal salvation in the hope that someone will be interested enough to offer lecturing work in a related area. During the last few years of studying, he has worked as a part-time lecturer in philosophy at Westminster College in Oxford, has been co-director of an educational conference company, has served as co-organizer of an international series of conferences on "evil," and has set up "The Marian Shrines Project" which aims to produce a comprehensive historical guide to Shrines of "Our Lady" in England and Wales. Outside of academic work, Day is involved with the Church, enjoys music and furniture, and dreams of Lambretta scooters and kit cars.

Anne Eyre, Coventry University, UK. Eyre has a Ph.D. in the Sociology of Religion from the University of Liverpool. She is an active member of the International Society for the Sociology of Religion and the British Sociological Association's Religion Study Group. She developed an interest in the culture, beliefs, and practices of Chinese, Malay, and Indian communities in South East Asia while lecturing in West Malaysia for two years. She has maintained an interest in the Sociology of Death and Dying and, more specifically, in the Sociology of Disasters, since returning to Britain. She currently lectures at Coventry University's Center for Disaster Management in Disaster Studies.

Gavin J. Fairbairn, University of Glenmorgan, Wales, UK. Fairbairn, Ph.D., is currently Professor of Professional Development in Nursing and Midwifery, following a career in special education, social work, and teacher education. He has developed interests in academic literacy and other aspects of education, in relation to which he has published many articles. He was also the author, with

Chris Winch, of *Reading, Writing, and Reasoning* (Open University Press, 2nd ed., 1996), and, with Susan Fairbairn, of *Reading at University* (Open University Press, 2001). His work in applied philosophy and professional ethics has included many articles, chapters, and several books, including *Contemplating Suicide, The Language and Ethics of Self Harm* (Routledge, 1995) and, with Denis Rowley and Maggie Bowen, of *Sexuality, Learning Difficulties, and Doing What's Right* (David Fulton Ltd, 1995).

Robert N. Fisher, Oxford, UK. Fisher is interested in all aspects of evil, suffering, pain, illness, disease, death, holocaust, and genocide. As the former Head of Theology and Principal Lecturer in Philosophy, Theology, and Theodicy at Westminster College, Oxford, he became known as the source of all suffering in the College! His research in the area of Philosophical Theology led to his dissertation at the University of Oxford entitled: "The World and God: A Theology of Persons in Relationship." The title underlies his other main interest: persons. He is the founder of the Global Association for the Study of Persons, a member of the Steering Committee for the International Forum on Persons, on the Advisory Board for Essays in Personalist Studies, and a member of the Communitarian Forum. He presently runs his own company, Learning Solutions, and is an educational consultant. He is married to Fiona and has three children, three cats, and a fanatical interest in science fiction, Star Trek, and American Football.

John P. Lizza, Kutztown University, USA. Lizza is Associate Professor of Philosophy and Chair of the Department of Philosophy at Kutztown University in Pennsylvania, USA and an Adjunct Associate at The Hastings Center in Garrison, New York. His areas of specialization include philosophy of mind, and bio-ethics with concentrations involving persons, personal identity, and death. He has published numerous articles in various journals such as *Theoretical Medicine and Bioethics*, *Philosophy of Medicine*, and *The British Journal for the Philosophy of Science*. He is also working on a book on *Persons and Death*.

Reverend Margaret J. Morris, Leicestershire, UK. Morris is a non-stipendiary Anglican priest in the Diocese of Leicester and an honorary canon of Leicester Cathedral. She is the Bishop's Chaplain for People Affected by HIV. The community-based Chaplaincy project offers pastoral, spiritual, and practical support to people affected by HIV, their partners, families, friends, caretakers, and colleagues, irrespective of whether a person identifies with a particular religious tradition or not. Through friendship and partnership, Morris is committed to encouraging faith communities to break the silence around HIV, support those affected by it, and prevent the transmission of it. Since 1987, she has been actively involved in local, national, and international responses to HIV. Leicester is a religiously, culturally, and ethnically diverse city in the Midlands region of the UK. Many communities have strong ties with countries which have a high prevalence for HIV. Morris's main areas of interest are the vulnerability of women worldwide to HIV infection, the impact of religion on responses to the virus, and the people affected by it. Her M.Th. dissertation explored the role of religion in the implementation of Public Health Medicine's strategic responses to HIV. She is married with a son, a daughter, and a grand-daughter.

David A. Pailin, Manchester University, UK. Pailin, born 1936, studied history and then divinity at Trinity College, Cambridge. He studied theology at the Perkins School of Theology, Southern Methodist University, Dallas, USA and at Manchester University. He has taught the philosophy of religion at Manchester University since 1966. In 1979 and 1980, he was Dean of the Faculty of Theology, and from August 1994 to August 1997 he was Head of the Department of Philosophy. His books include *The Way to Faith* (a study of Newman's *Grammar of Assent*), *Attitudes to Other Religions, Comparative Religion in Seventeenth and Eighteenth-Century Britain, Groundwork of Philosophy of Religion, God and the Process of Reality, The Anthropological Character of Theology, The Gentle Touch: From a Theology of Handicap to a Theology of Human Being,* and *Probing the Foundations*. He has also contributed to a number of books and published articles in professional journals. He is currently working on a book on the use of resources and truth, reason debates in Britain from Herbert of Cherbury to William Paley. In connection with this, he collects seventeenth and eighteenth-century works on philosophy. He has two children and, to date, four grandchildren, who teach him many things that they think he does not know or remember.

Daniel T. Primozic, Elmhurst College, USA. Primozic, Chairperson and Associate Professor of Philosophy at Elmhurst College, has written a wide range of articles, almost all of which pertain to personhood, humanity, and the moral community. He is also the editor of *Dialogue,* the international journal of *Phi Sigma Tau*, has published *On Merleau-Ponty* (2000), and is currently writing *On C. S. Lewis*, both for the Wadsworth Philosopher Series.

Patricia Sayre, Saint Mary's College, USA. Sayre is most interested in questions that relate to issues of our lives. Her thinking about these issues owes a great deal to the work of Ludwig Wittgenstein, as well as to her joint classroom endeavors with her colleague Linnea Vacca. Such endeavors have provided an excellent opportunity to marry her love for literature to her compulsion to philosophize.

Eric O. Springsted, Princeton University, USA. Springsted teaches theology at Princeton and is formerly Professor of Religion, and Chaplain at Illinois College in Jacksonville, Illinois. After doing his undergraduate work at St. John's College, he received his divinity degree and doctorate in philosophy and theology from Princeton Theological Seminary. He is the author and editor of six books, including four on the French philosopher, Simone Weil. Co-founder of the American Weil Society, he has served as its President since 1981. He has written on education, theology, culture, and the philosophy of religion. He is a member of the Center of Theological Inquiry in Princeton, and is currently working on a book on the nature of faith and the nature of the self, as well as editing an anthology of Weil's spiritual writings and a volume of essays on spirituality and theology.

Joel A. Thompson, University of St. Andrews, UK. Thompson is a graduate of Elmhurst College, having received a B.A. in Philosophy in 2000. His post-graduate work began at the University of St. Andrews for an M.Litt degree in Philosophy. His areas of interests include philosophy of mind, moral philosophy and ethics, decision theory, and philosophical Taoism. He is a member of *Phi Sigma Tau* (the International Philosophy Honor Society), *Phi Kappa Phi*, and a student member of the American Philosophical Practioners Association.

Linnea Vacca, Saint Mary's College, USA. Linnea Vacca teaches literature and women's studies at Saint Mary's College in Notre Dame, Indiana, USA. She spends her spring semesters teaching Italian literature in the Saint Mary's Rome Program and taking full advantage of the Mediterranean sun. She is currently working on a book with Patricia Sayre that examines the problem of other minds from a moral and literary perspective.

Index

VIBS

The **Value Inquiry Book Series** is co-sponsored by:

Adler School of Professional Psychology
American Indian Philosophy Association
American Maritain Association
American Society for Value Inquiry
Association for Process Philosophy of Education
Canadian Society for Philosophical Practice
Center for Bioethics, University of Turku
Center for Professional and Applied Ethics, University of North Carolina at Charlotte
Center for Research in Cognitive Science, Autonomous University of Barcelona
Centre for Applied Ethics, Hong Kong Baptist University
Centre for Cultural Research, Aarhus University
Centre for Professional Ethics, University of Central Lancashire
Centre for the Study of Philosophy and Religion, University College of Cape Breton
College of Education and Allied Professions, Bowling Green State University
College of Liberal Arts, Rochester Institute of Technology
Concerned Philosophers for Peace
Conference of Philosophical Societies
Department of Moral and Social Philosophy, University of Helsinki
Gannon University
Gilson Society
Ikeda University
Institute of Philosophy of the High Council of Scientific Research, Spain
International Academy of Philosophy of the Principality of Liechtenstein
International Association of Bioethics
International Center for the Arts, Humanities, and Value Inquiry
International Society for Universal Dialogue
Natural Law Society
Personalist Discussion Group
Philosophical Society of Finland
Philosophy Born of Struggle Association
Philosophy Seminar, University of Mainz
Pragmatism Archive
R.S. Hartman Institute for Formal and Applied Axiology
Research Institute, Lakeridge Health Corporation
Russian Philosophical Society
Society for Iberian and Latin-American Thought
Society for the Philosophic Study of Genocide and the Holocaust
Society for the Philosophy of Sex and Love
Yves R. Simon Institute

Titles Published

1. Noel Balzer, *The Human Being as a Logical Thinker*

2. Archie J. Bahm, *Axiology: The Science of Values*

3. H. P. P. (Hennie) Lötter, *Justice for an Unjust Society*

4. H. G. Callaway, *Context for Meaning and Analysis: A Critical Study in the Philosophy of Language*

5. Benjamin S. Llamzon, *A Humane Case for Moral Intuition*

6. James R. Watson, *Between Auschwitz and Tradition: Postmodern Reflections on the Task of Thinking.* A volume in **Holocaust and Genocide Studies**

7. Robert S. Hartman, *Freedom to Live: The Robert Hartman Story, edited by Arthur R. Ellis.* A volume in **Hartman Institute Axiology Studies**

8. Archie J. Bahm, *Ethics: The Science of Oughtness*

9. George David Miller, *An Idiosyncratic Ethics; Or, the Lauramachean Ethics*

10. Joseph P. DeMarco, *A Coherence Theory in Ethics*

11. Frank G. Forrest, *Valuemetrics℠: The Science of Personal and Professional Ethics.* A volume in **Hartman Institute Axiology Studies**

12. William Gerber, *The Meaning of Life: Insights of the World's Great Thinkers*

13. Richard T. Hull, Editor, *A Quarter Century of Value Inquiry: Presidential Addresses of the American Society for Value Inquiry.* A volume in **Histories and Addresses of Philosophical Societies**

14. William Gerber, *Nuggets of Wisdom from Great Jewish Thinkers: From Biblical Times to the Present*

15. Sidney Axinn, *The Logic of Hope: Extensions of Kant's View of Religion*

16. Messay Kebede, *Meaning and Development*

17. Amihud Gilead, *The Platonic Odyssey: A Philosophical-Literary Inquiry into the Phaedo*

18. Necip Fikri Alican, *Mill's Principle of Utility: A Defense of John Stuart Mill's Notorious Proof.* A volume in **Universal Justice**

19. Michael H. Mitias, Editor, *Philosophy and Architecture.*

20. Roger T. Simonds, *Rational Individualism: The Perennial Philosophy of Legal Interpretation.* A volume in **Natural Law Studies**

21. William Pencak, *The Conflict of Law and Justice in the Icelandic Sagas*

22. Samuel M. Natale and Brian M. Rothschild, Editors, *Values, Work, Education: The Meanings of Work*

23. N. Georgopoulos and Michael Heim, Editors, *Being Human in the Ultimate: Studies in the Thought of John M. Anderson*

24. Robert Wesson and Patricia A. Williams, Editors, *Evolution and Human Values*

25. Wim J. van der Steen, *Facts, Values, and Methodology: A New Approach to Ethics*

26. Avi Sagi and Daniel Statman, *Religion and Morality*

27. Albert William Levi, *The High Road of Humanity: The Seven Ethical Ages of Western Man*, Edited by Donald Phillip Verene and Molly Black Verene

28. Samuel M. Natale and Brian M. Rothschild, Editors, *Work Values: Education, Organization, and Religious Concerns*

29. Laurence F. Bove and Laura Duhan Kaplan, Editors, From the Eye of the Storm: Regional Conflicts and the Philosophy of Peace. A volume in **Philosophy of Peace**

30. Robin Attfield, *Value, Obligation, and Meta-Ethics*

31. William Gerber, *The Deepest Questions You Can Ask About God: As Answered by the World's Great Thinkers*

32. Daniel Statman, *Moral Dilemmas*

33. Rem B. Edwards, Editor, *Formal Axiology and Its Critics.* A volume in **Hartman Institute Axiology Studies**

34. George David Miller and Conrad P. Pritscher, *On Education and Values: In Praise of Pariahs and Nomads.* A volume in **Philosophy of Education**

35. Paul S. Penner, *Altruistic Behavior: An Inquiry into Motivation*

36. Corbin Fowler, *Morality for Moderns*

37. Giambattista Vico, *The Art of Rhetoric* (*Institutiones Oratoriae*, 1711–1741), from the definitive Latin text and notes, Italian commentary and introduction by Giuliano Crifò. Translated and Edited by Giorgio A. Pinton and Arthur W. Shippee. A volume in **Values in Italian Philosophy**

38. W. H. Werkmeister, *Martin Heidegger on the Way*. Edited by Richard T. Hull. A volume in **Werkmeister Studies**

39. Phillip Stambovsky, *Myth and the Limits of Reason*

40. Samantha Brennan, Tracy Isaacs, and Michael Milde, Editors, *A Question of Values: New Canadian Perspectives in Ethics and Political Philosophy*

41. Peter A. Redpath, *Cartesian Nightmare: An Introduction to Transcendental Sophistry*. A volume in **Studies in the History of Western Philosophy**

42. Clark Butler, *History as the Story of Freedom: Philosophy in Intercultural Context*, with responses by sixteen scholars

43. Dennis Rohatyn, *Philosophy History Sophistry*

44. Leon Shaskolsky Sheleff, *Social Cohesion and Legal Coercion: A Critique of Weber, Durkheim, and Marx*. Afterword by Virginia Black

45. Alan Soble, Editor, *Sex, Love, and Friendship: Studies of the Society for the Philosophy of Sex and Love, 1977–1992*. A volume **in Histories and Addresses of Philosophical Societies**

46. Peter A. Redpath, *Wisdom's Odyssey: From Philosophy to Transcendental Sophistry*. A volume in **Studies in the History of Western Philosophy**

47. Albert A. Anderson, *Universal Justice: A Dialectical Approach*. A volume in **Universal Justice**

48. Pio Colonnello, *The Philosophy of José Gaos*. Translated from Italian by Peter Cocozzella. Edited by Myra Moss. Introduction by Giovanni Gullace. A volume in **Values in Italian Philosophy**

49. Laura Duhan Kaplan and Laurence F. Bove, Editors, *Philosophical Perspectives on Power and Domination: Theories and Practices*. A volume in **Philosophy of Peace**

50. Gregory F. Mellema, *Collective Responsibility*

51. Josef Seifert, *What Is Life? The Originality, Irreducibility, and Value of Life*. A volume in **Central-European Value Studies**

52. William Gerber, *Anatomy of What We Value Most*

53. Armando Molina, *Our Ways: Values and Character*, Edited by Rem B. Edwards. A volume in **Hartman Institute Axiology Studies**

54. Kathleen J. Wininger, *Nietzsche's Reclamation of Philosophy*. A volume in **Central-European Value Studies**

55. Thomas Magnell, Editor, *Explorations of Value*

56. HPP (Hennie) Lötter, *Injustice, Violence, and Peace: The Case of South Africa*. A volume in **Philosophy of Peace**

57. Lennart Nordenfelt, *Talking About Health: A Philosophical Dialogue*. A volume in **Nordic Value Studies**

58. Jon Mills and Janusz A. Polanowski, *The Ontology of Prejudice*. A volume in **Philosophy and Psychology**

59. Leena Vilkka, *The Intrinsic Value of Nature*

60. Palmer Talbutt, Jr., Rough Dialectics: *Sorokin's Philosophy of Value*, with contributions by Lawrence T. Nichols and Pitirim A. Sorokin

61. C. L. Sheng, *A Utilitarian General Theory of Value*

62. George David Miller, *Negotiating Toward Truth: The Extinction of Teachers and Students*. Epilogue by Mark Roelof Eleveld. A volume in **Philosophy of Education**

63. William Gerber, *Love, Poetry, and Immortality: Luminous Insights of the World's Great Thinkers*

64. Dane R. Gordon, Editor, *Philosophy in Post-Communist Europe*. A volume in **Post-Communist European Thought**

65. Dane R. Gordon and Józef Niznik, Editors, *Criticism and Defense of Rationality in Contemporary Philosophy*. A volume in **Post-Communist European Thought**

66. John R. Shook, *Pragmatism: An Annotated Bibliography, 1898-1940*. With contributions by E. Paul Colella, Lesley Friedman, Frank X. Ryan, and Ignas K. Skrupskelis

67. Lansana Keita, *The Human Project and the Temptations of Science*

68. Michael M. Kazanjian, *Phenomenology and Education: Cosmology, Co-Being, and Core Curriculum*. A volume in **Philosophy of Education**

69. James W. Vice, *The Reopening of the American Mind: On Skepticism and Constitutionalism*

70. Sarah Bishop Merrill, *Defining Personhood: Toward the Ethics of Quality in Clinical Care*

71. Dane R. Gordon, *Philosophy and Vision*

72. Alan Milchman and Alan Rosenberg, Editors, *Postmodernism and the Holocaust*. A volume in **Holocaust and Genocide Studies**

73. Peter A. Redpath, *Masquerade of the Dream Walkers: Prophetic Theology from the Cartesians to Hegel*. A volume in **Studies in the History of Western Philosophy**

74. Malcolm D. Evans, *Whitehead and Philosophy of Education: The Seamless Coat of Learning*. A volume in **Philosophy of Education**

75. Warren E. Steinkraus, *Taking Religious Claims Seriously: A Philosophy of Religion*, edited by Michael H. Mitias. A volume in **Universal Justice**

76. Thomas Magnell, Editor, *Values and Education*

77. Kenneth A. Bryson, *Persons and Immortality*. A volume in **Natural Law Studies**

78. Steven V. Hicks, *International Law and the Possibility of a Just World Order: An Essay on Hegel's Universalism*. A volume in **Universal Justice**

79. E. F. Kaelin, *Texts on Texts and Textuality: A Phenomenology of Literary Art*, Edited by Ellen J. Burns

80. Amihud Gilead, Saving Possibilities: A Study in Philosophical Psychology. *A volume in Philosophy and Psychology*

81. André Mineau, *The Making of the Holocaust: Ideology and Ethics in the Systems Perspective*. A volume in **Holocaust and Genocide Studies**

82. Howard P. Kainz, *Politically Incorrect Dialogues: Topics Not Discussed in Polite Circles*

83. Veikko Launis, Juhani Pietarinen, and Juha Räikkä, Editors, *Genes and Morality: New Essays*. A volume in **Nordic Value Studies**

84. Steven Schroeder, *The Metaphysics of Cooperation: A Study of F. D. Maurice*

85. Caroline Joan ("Kay") S. Picart, *Thomas Mann and Friedrich Nietzsche: Eroticism, Death, Music, and Laughter*. A volume in **Central-European Value Studies**

86. G. John M. Abbarno, Editor, *The Ethics of Homelessness: Philosophical Perspectives*

87. James Giles, Editor, *French Existentialism: Consciousness, Ethics, and Relations with Others*. A volume in **Nordic Value Studies**

88. Deane Curtin and Robert Litke, Editors, *Institutional Violence*. A volume in **Philosophy of Peace**

89. Yuval Lurie, *Cultural Beings: Reading the Philosophers of Genesis*

90. Sandra A. Wawrytko, Editor, *The Problem of Evil: An Intercultural Exploration*. A volume in **Philosophy and Psychology**

91. Gary J. Acquaviva, *Values, Violence, and Our Future*. A volume in **Hartman Institute Axiology Studies**

92. Michael R. Rhodes, *Coercion: A Nonevaluative Approach*

93. Jacques Kriel, *Matter, Mind, and Medicine: Transforming the Clinical Method*

94. Haim Gordon, *Dwelling Poetically: Educational Challenges in Heidegger's Thinking on Poetry*. A volume in **Philosophy of Education**

95. Ludwig Grünberg, *The Mystery of Values: Studies in Axiology*, edited by Cornelia Grünberg and Laura Grünberg

96. Gerhold K. Becker, Editor, *The Moral Status of Persons: Perspectives on Bioethics*. A volume in **Studies in Applied Ethics**

97. Roxanne Claire Farrar, *Sartrean Dialectics: A Method for Critical Discourse on Aesthetic Experience*

98. Ugo Spirito, *Memoirs of the Twentieth Century*. Translated from Italian and edited by Anthony G. Costantini. A volume in **Values in Italian Philosophy**

99. Steven Schroeder, *Between Freedom and Necessity: An Essay on the Place of Value*

100. Foster N. Walker, *Enjoyment and the Activity of Mind: Dialogues on Whitehead and Education*. A volume in **Philosophy of Education**

101. Avi Sagi, Kierkegaard, *Religion, and Existence: The Voyage of the Self*. Translated from Hebrew by Batya Stein

102. Bennie R. Crockett, Jr., Editor, *Addresses of the Mississippi Philosophical Association*. A volume in **Histories and Addresses of Philosophical Societies**

103. Paul van Dijk, *Anthropology in the Age of Technology: The Philosophical Contribution of Günther Anders*

104. Giambattista Vico, *Universal Right*. Translated from Latin and Edited by Giorgio Pinton and Margaret Diehl. A volume in **Values in Italian Philosophy**

105. Judith Presler and Sally J. Scholz, Editors, *Peacemaking: Lessons from the Past, Visions for the Future*. A volume in **Philosophy of Peace**

106. Dennis Bonnette, *Origin of the Human Species*. A volume in **Studies in the History of Western Philosophy**

107. Phyllis Chiasson, *Peirce's Pragmatism: The Design for Thinking*. A volume in **Studies in Pragmatism and Values**

108. Dan Stone, Editor, *Theoretical Interpretations of the Hol*ocaust. A volume in **Holocaust and Genocide Studies**

109. Raymond Angelo Belliotti, *What Is the Meaning of Human Life?*

110. Lennart Nordenfelt, *Health, Science, and Ordinary Language*, with Contributions by George Khushf and K. W. M. Fulford

111. Daryl Koehn, *Local Insights, Global Ethics for Business*. A volume in **Studies in Applied Ethics**

112. Matti Häyry and Tuija Takala, Editors, *The Future of Value Inquiry*. A volume in **Nordic Value Studies**

113. Conrad P. Pritscher, *Quantum Learning: Beyond Duality*

114. Thomas M. Dicken and Rem B. Edwards, *Dialogues on Values and Centers of Value: Old Friends, New Thoughts*. A volume in **Hartman Institute Axiology Studies**

115. Rem B. Edwards, *What Caused the Big Bang?* A volume in **Philosophy and Religion**

116. Jon Mills, Editor, *A Pedagogy of Becoming*. A volume in **Philosophy of Education**

117. Robert T. Radford, *Cicero: A Study in the Origins of Republican Philosophy*. A volume in **Studies in the History of Western Philosophy**

118. Arleen L. F. Salles and María Julia Bertomeu, Editors, *Bioethics: Latin American Perspectives*. A volume in **Philosophy in Latin America**

119. Nicola Abbagnano, *The Human Project: The Year 2000*, with an Interview by Guiseppe Grieco. Translated from Italian by Bruno Martini and Nino Langiulli. Edited with an introduction by Nino Langiulli. A volume in **Studies in the History of Western Philosophy**

120. Daniel M. Haybron, Editor, *Earth's Abominations: Philosophical Studies of Evil*. A volume in **Personalist Studies**

121. Anna T. Challenger, *Philosophy and Art in Gurdjieff's Beelzebub: A Modern Sufi Odyssey*

122. George David Miller, *Peace, Value, and Wisdom: The Educational Philosophy of Daisaku Ikeda*. A volume in **Daisaku Ikeda Studies**

123. Haim Gordon and Rivca Gordon, *Sophistry and Twentieth-Century Art*

124. Thomas O Buford and Harold H. Oliver, Editors *Personalism Revisited: Its Proponents and Critics*. A volume in **Histories and Addresses of Philosophical Societies**

125. Avi Sagi, *Albert Camus and the Philosophy of the Absurd*. Translated from Hebrew by Batya Stein

126. Robert S. Hartman, *The Knowledge of Good: Critique of Axiologic l Reason*. Expanded translation from the Spanish by Robert S. Hartman. Edited by Arthur R. Ellis and Rem B. Edwards. A volume in **Hartman Institute Axiology Studies**

127. Alison Bailey and Paula J. Smithka, Editors. *Community, Diversity, and Difference: Implications for Peace*. A volume in **Philosophy of Peace**

128. Oscar Vilarroya, *The Dissolution of Mind: A Fable of How Experience Gives Rise to Cognition.* A volume in **Cognitive Science**

129. Paul Bube and Jefferey Geller, Editors, *Conversations with Pragmatism.* A volume in **Studies in Pragmatism and Values**

130. Richard Rumana, *Richard Rorty: An Annotated Bibliography of Secondary Literature.* A volume in **Studies in Pragmatism and Values**

131. Stephen Schneck, *Max Scheler's Acting Persons: New Perspectives.* A volume in **Personalist Studies**

132. Michael Kazanjian, *Learning Values Lifelong: From Inert Ideas to Wholes.* A volume in **Philosophy of Education**

133. Rudolph Alexander Kofi Cain: *Alain Leroy Locke: Race, Culture, and the Education of African American Adults.* A Volume in **African American Philosophy.**

134. Werner J. Krieglstein, *Compassion: A New Philosophy of the Other.*

135. Robert N. Fisher, Daniel T. Primozic, Peter A. Day, and Joel A. Thompson, Editors, *Suffering, Death, and Identity.* A volume in **Personalist Studies**